# SuperLife

# SuperLife

THE 5 SIMPLE FIXES
THAT WILL MAKE YOU
HEALTHY, FIT, AND
ETERNALLY AWESOME

## Darin Olien

**HARPER** WAVE

*An Imprint of* HarperCollins*Publishers*

This book contains advice and information relating to health care. It should be used to supplement rather than replace the advice of your doctor or another trained health professional. If you know or suspect you have a health problem, it is recommended that you seek your physician's advice before embarking on any medical program or treatment. All efforts have been made to assure the accuracy of the information contained in this book as of the date of publication. This publisher and the author disclaim liability for any medical outcomes that may occur as a result of applying the methods suggested in this book.

HarperCollins books may be purchased for educational, business, or sales promotional use. For information, please e-mail the Special Markets Department at SPsales@harpercollins.com.

A hardcover edition of this book was published in 2015 by Harper Wave, an imprint of HarperCollins Publishers.

FIRST HARPER WAVE PAPERBACK EDITION PUBLISHED 2017

Library of Congress Cataloging-in-Publication Data has been applied for.

ISBN: 978-0-06-229719-8 (pbk.)

17  18  19  20  21      OV/RRD      10  9  8  7  6  5  4  3  2  1

*To my late father,*
*who always encouraged and supported me*
*in the face of adversity, and to my mother, who forever*
*nurtured and loved me as I found my way*

# Contents

# Introduction

I'm really psyched.

But before I explain why, I want to tell you about when I saw the comedian Louis CK on one of the late-night talk shows.

He'd just been on a plane, he said, when the attendant announced that Wi-Fi service was now available. The guy sitting next to him immediately began working away on his laptop, but after a few minutes the Wi-Fi suddenly went off.

"This is bullshit!" the guy said angrily.

Louis CK said he immediately thought, here we are sitting in chairs that fly through the air at five hundred miles an hour, and this guy is pissed because he can't read his e-mail?

That's funny and brilliant because it's so true—about all of us. We become so accustomed to the miracles that surround us every day, we don't even notice them.

I'm talking about your body. My body, too. Everybody's body.

It's a freaking miracle. Not just one miracle, either—it's an infinite number of freaking miracles.

It's so mind-boggling that we can hardly begin to grasp it all. If we really had to stop and think about every amazing, breathtaking, jaw-dropping thing that our bodies are constantly doing, completely on their own and without any conscious effort on our part, without us even knowing about it, we wouldn't have time to do anything else. We'd be too dazzled to try.

Turning water into wine is a miracle, no doubt. But is it more miraculous than turning broccoli, walnuts, beets, apples, and water into bones and organs and blood and brains? Not to me.

I started writing this book when I was thirteen years old.

I was sitting on the living room floor back home in Minnesota, eating my Cocoa Puffs and watching cartoons. Next thing I remember, somebody was talking about the grapefruit diet and how it made them feel fantastic and healthier than they had ever been before.

I began paying very close attention.

At this point in my life, I was a mess. I had been born prematurely, weighed 3.5 pounds and was given a fifty-fifty chance of surviving. I made it, but with underdeveloped lungs and a lot of other difficulties. By second grade I wore glasses and a patch over one eye and had severe headaches, a resting heart rate of 120 beats per minute—about the same as a hummingbird's—a bad case of hyperactivity, and some kind of thyroid problem, which they medicated with a pharmaceutical cocktail. By the age of ten I had water on my knees and had undergone various medical treatments for allergies and immune system dysfunction and other weirdness. I was removed from the normal kids' classroom due to what the doctors and teachers believed were learning disabilities.

I was a wreck.

After the commercial ended, I put down my Cocoa Puffs and asked my mother to buy me some grapefruit—a lot of it. I began eating it for breakfast and several other times a day. The grapefruit replaced the pizza, candy, soda, and all the rest of the junk I had been pouring into my body.

I started to feel different. Better. Making my own decisions, ones that worked, empowered me. I stopped taking my hyperactivity pills too. I didn't tell anybody. I just did it. That made me feel even better. Cooler.

Of course I didn't stay on the grapefruit diet permanently. I reverted to the sketchy eating routine of a normal midwestern kid. But as I grew up, I continued paying close attention to what I ate and drank and how it made me feel.

I've been on this path—trying things and getting feedback—

ever since. I'm not a professional scientist—I'm an eternal student. But I've learned a lot along the way, and I'm constantly discovering more.

I became an athlete in high school and played football in college. A back injury eventually ended my career, but my passion for learning about what makes us healthy was stronger than ever. I studied exercise physiology and nutrition in college, worked one-on-one helping people who were injured, discovered more about what makes our bodies tick. I read everything I could get my hands on, and then I went out to meet scientists and researchers who were devoting their lives to the study of health and nutrition, and picked their brains.

When an expert told me something that made sense, I tried it out on myself. If I felt better, I stuck with it. If I didn't, I moved on. I read lots of scholarly papers, but I didn't wait around for experts to tell me what to do. I jumped in and figured it out on my own.

I went from thirteen-year-old wreck to college football player to nutrition counselor and physical trainer, and now I spend my time traveling around the world investigating and searching for the most intensely powerful foods, the healthiest, most amazingly nutritious things that nature has ever made. Superfood Hunter is the title that's stuck, but my passion for this subject goes so much farther and deeper than that.

Now I'm psyched because I get the chance to tell you everything I've learned about our bodies, what they need, and how they really operate.

Like this: disease doesn't exist.

I know how insane that sounds, but it's true. Disease doesn't exist. At least not how it's been explained to us by doctors and scientists.

Here's how we've been taught to think: We go through life feeling fine, with fingers crossed, hoping we always stay that way, but knowing that at some point something bad is going to happen. Something's going to break down. Something's going to go haywire. Maybe it will be our hearts, or our livers, or our blood, our lungs, our colons, our bones, our brains, our breasts. Someday, something will go wrong.

And then it does. Dammit! Why me?

Now we have a disease. It's probably got a scary name. There's usually a specialist nearby who treats nothing else. If we're lucky, it's something the doctors and pharmacists can fix. Otherwise, we may be in real trouble.

According to what we've been taught by the experts, that's disease. Except it's not.

If we're worrying about our heart or our head or our prostate or our pancreas or our kidneys or anything like that, we're already looking at the wrong thing. We're working with bad information.

We're not paying attention to what really matters.

All those "diseases"—they're just symptoms. They are signs that something has been allowed to go wrong inside us. Once the symptoms get bad enough, they become genuine problems, true. But even when we treat them, we're still dealing only with the symptom. Not the underlying cause.

Here's what I've learned: every disease has many possible little causes, but the little causes are all the result of just a few big causes. We keep treating the little causes, and they keep on happening. If instead we deal with the big causes, then suddenly disease becomes something we can prevent rather than just treat.

I'm talking about every sickness, especially the seriously gnarly ones, the modern-day terrors that either end our lives too soon or leave us alive but sickly and infirm for years, decades. Chronic ailments like diabetes, emphysema, arthritis, heart disease, cancer . . .

The truth is, we're not supposed to get sick at all. And if we do, we're meant to recover fully and fast. We're built to be amazing physical beings, each one of us. Our bodies are genetically programmed to be healthy and lively and strong. When we do become ill, it's unnatural, not inevitable.

Our number-one killer, heart disease—mostly preventable.

Our number-two killer, cancer—the same. Believe it or not, there are places on this planet where those two scourges are uncommon. But here, where we enjoy the most expensive and scientifically advanced medical care in the world, they are everyday tragedies.

I'm always amazed when I ask people how they're doing, and their answer goes something like this: *Oh, I'm OK. No complaints. Just the usual little aches and pains. My knees hurt sometimes. My back, too. I get these headaches once in a while. I've always had trouble falling asleep at night, and then by the middle of the afternoon I'm fighting to stay awake. A little heartburn occasionally. Constipated now and then. Wish I still had the same old energy in the sack, but who does? Just the normal stuff, like everybody else . . .*

*What?* I want to yell. You think that's normal? We're not meant to have *any* of those complaints. We're built to feel great—full of energy and life. No headaches or backaches or stomachaches, no weariness, no digestive system distress. No uninspired sex. No joyless existence. We've somehow accepted that this is what it's like to be an adult. Wrong!

So many people feel just slightly lousy and still think they're doing OK. Isn't OK good enough? You know what? This is the only lifetime we're getting, and OK is definitely not good enough.

In fact, all those little complaints are really early warning signals of something seriously bad in the future. Constipation today, colon cancer tomorrow. Insomnia now, a major heart attack someday. Even erectile dysfunction—by treating it with pills we mask the causes, but if blood vessels in the penis have narrowed, it means that arteries elsewhere are closing off, too. A limp dick tonight, a stroke down the line.

We'll discuss all that and more, but for now I just want you to think about this: by our actions, we determine our fate. Health or sickness? Joy or misery? Pain or pleasure? Life or death? Largely up to us.

All those big, bad, scary diseases? We invite them in or we shut them out. That can be a heavy burden, I realize. But it's also a great freedom to determine how healthy we will be. Either way, it all depends on whether we did or did not take care of something important.

That's what this whole book is all about. The something important.

I want to help people take responsibility for the one thing we will have from when we are born until we die. I want us all to take what nature has given us and use it to the fullest, and for the longest time possible. Not just go through life accepting whatever comes along, waiting for that bad thing to happen. Because we can do a lot to prevent ill health, and we can feel great as we do it. I want us all to be open to the possibility of feeling amazing every day.

It starts with the beautiful freaking miracle that carries us through our lives from start to finish—our bodies.

*Part One*

# The 5 Life Forces

# What Are the Five Life Forces?

*And Why Do They Matter So Much?*

I probably should have mentioned this before: I'm giving everyone who reads this book a Ferrari.

That's right, a beautiful top-of-the-line, world-class precision machine just for the price of a book. Of course there's a catch: you have to take care of it. That means the right kind of fuel. The proper treatment. And you need to drive it the way it was meant to be driven.

Do all that, though, and the Ferrari is yours.

Actually, it's already yours, though it may feel more like a rusted-out junker than a high-performance work of automotive art. But somewhere inside each of us is a human body that can operate and respond like a Ferrari.

I'm going to give you your Ferrari by providing you with the operating manual they neglected to include back when you were born. Because how can you take care of yourself properly if you don't know what makes you run right? You can't.

My operating manual is a lot simpler than the booklet that comes with a fancy Italian car, trust me.

You only need to pay attention to five things to control what kind of health you'll enjoy. That's right—just five factors that determine whether you will be strong and vital and fit and happy, or if you will be sickly and infirm and out of shape and miserable. Whether you will age well or badly, or at all.

Five factors.

The word *factors* is kind of boring, but the scientific world hasn't come up with a term yet for exactly what I'm talking about. So let's just call them what they truly are: life forces.

Five life forces—the only things that control our health. The only things we need to think about.

It's like they say about money—if we take care of the pennies, the dollars take care of themselves. Take care of the five life forces, and our bodies will do the rest. That's what our bodies were made to do.

The life forces are:

NUTRITION. Pretty straightforward, right? It means everything we eat. The foods themselves, and also everything they contain, which can be a very long list. We may not always know everything that's on that list, but our bodies do.

HYDRATION. The mere fact that we are mostly water should be enough to explain this one.

OXYGENATION. Like water, we know we need it, though we don't all know the many reasons why.

ALKALIZATION. This one's a bit trickier. It has to do with the balance of acidity and alkalinity of our internal environment.

DETOXIFICATION. This includes our immune system, which has a lot to deal with, plus the process of handling all the toxins and poisons and other junk the world throws at us.

That's all of it.

We've been taught to think of our blood and organs and bones and nerves and skin and everything else as separate matters, each of which comes with different issues and concerns. But the truth is that every single thing in our bodies, every molecule and cell, responds to those five life forces.

The medical world has organized itself by specialty—one doctor treats the brain, another our feet, our hearts, our endocrine systems, and each comes up with its own rules and regulations. But the same internal conditions that affect our brains also affect our feet, our skin, our genitals, and our joints. The internal environment we create is identical for our livers, our immune systems, our stomachs, and our eyeballs. We are made up of around 70 trillion cells, and they all have the same basic needs.

We just have to understand what those needs are—the five life forces. And then we have to fix the way we fulfill them. That's right. Five simple fixes stand between you and feeling healthy, fit, and eternally awesome.

Let's talk about how.

# Life Force Number One:
# Nutrition

Nutrition is a great, important subject. It's truly the cornerstone of health. There's no better place to begin a discussion of the five life forces.

But I'd much rather talk about eating.

Eating is the most intimate thing we will ever do, and I know what you're thinking, but eating is even more intimate than that, and I'll tell you why. When we eat, we open our bodies wide and expose ourselves, every single cell, to whatever's out there in our environment. It's how we turn the *out there* into the *in here*. When we eat, those external things actually become us. Our organs, bones, muscles, nerves, skin, blood, and everything else are made from what we eat and drink—there's nothing else to work with. Before we were born, we were completely created, cell by cell, by what our mothers ate and drank. Today, it's no different, except now we're the ones doing the eating and the drinking, inventing our bodies.

When we look in the mirror, that's what we see—all the things we've eaten. Want to know what shape you're in? Just think back to everything you consumed over the past week. There's your answer. Now, let's talk about the big, fresh, leafy green salad loaded with raw vegetables and nuts you had for lunch, or the organic berry smoothie you just made. Or was it a bacon double cheeseburger and a jelly doughnut or some other manufactured fake food, and some heavily sugared or—even worse—chemically sweetened carbonated liquid candy to wash it down?

Either way, ask yourself: Is this what I want to be made out of? Is this the being I want to be?

These questions are the beginning of all wisdom when it comes to nutrition—or, even better, eating.

Okay, so what should we eat?

A huge percentage of all the scientific research ever conducted has been devoted to answering that seemingly simple question. It's amazing how much brilliance and effort have to go into something so basic. *What am I supposed to eat?* How can it be that every beast, every fish, every insect—every other critter on the face of the planet—can figure this out so easily, and yet here we are, still wondering?

Maybe we just have too many choices.

Let's face it, we already know how we should eat. The problem is that we're too good at pretending we don't. It's the only way we could go on downing some of the junk we consume, stuff we know is doing us harm. No other animal does that.

I'm going to distill this entire book into a single sentence:

Eat a wide variety of whole, fresh, clean foods—mostly vegetables, fruit, beans, nuts, seeds, grains, sprouts, and healthy fats. Eat a lot of it raw.

Okay, it took me two sentences, but there! It's that simple. How can we pretend not to understand? I think maybe part of the problem is that it's *too* simple. There's no wiggle room. No loopholes. We either adopt it or ignore it.

Now you may have noticed that my description of what we should eat includes a conspicuous omission: animal foods, meaning meat, fish, eggs, and dairy products. It wasn't an accident. After a great deal of personal experience and study, I have reached the conclusion that the fewer of these foods we eat, the healthier we tend to be. But this isn't a blanket endorsement of the vegan route either. I used to eat meat, and I was real healthy.

Some people have a hard time getting all the nutrients they need from plant foods, and so for them some animal-based foods are a necessity. This would be a less complicated subject if meat, fish, and all the rest hadn't been turned into industrial products that often come with unhealthy, unnatural baggage. I'll discuss this in more detail in "The Protein Fat Myths," and the one on nutritional stress. But for now I want to keep the focus on the healthiest foods we can eat.

In 2013 the results of a major scientific trial of the so-called Mediterranean diet were published by the *New England Journal of Medicine*. Researchers from the University of Barcelona and elsewhere put over 7,000 adult subjects onto various eating plans; those on the typical Mediterranean diet offered definitive proof at last that if we eat leafy greens and lots of other vegetables, fruit, nuts, fish, and olive oil, everything fresh and unprocessed, and only a small amount of meat and dairy, we'll be healthier and enjoy greater longevity. In other words, they discovered that if we want to live long and well, we should eat like Greek grandmothers do. Those grandmothers could have told us the same thing for free, but would we have listened?

The same basic advice comes from Dr. Caldwell Esselstyn, formerly of the renowned Cleveland Clinic, and one of the world's most respected experts on the subject of cardiac health. He calls heart disease "a completely preventable food-borne illness."

If only we had known! Or did we? At any rate, once he made this pronouncement, which was widely reported, it became a lot harder to pretend ignorance. About 600,000 deaths a year in the United States alone. Almost all caused by lousy eating. Completely preventable.

A wide variety of whole, fresh, clean, mostly plant-based foods. Adopt or ignore?

# Feeding Our Cells

To understand why these are the keys to proper nutrition, we need to remind ourselves of something pretty basic: before we eat our food, our food eats.

It, too, is nourished; it grows up and develops; it absorbs and metabolizes and excretes and retains and makes use of what it needs.

What does food eat? Sunlight. Plants actually consume and store the energy of a star that's 93 million miles away, a pretty cool trick. Air. Water.

Mostly, though, it is nourished by the soil. What's in there? More than we imagine. Dirt is a mysterious, complex stew of minerals, vitamins, metals, organic materials, microbes—microscopic living organisms that themselves consume and excrete—and lots of other essential stuff. The plant, the tree, the vine, they take their nourishment from the soil and use it to grow their product—the produce—until we come along and eat it.

Not coincidentally—since we and those plants are all alive, an important thing to have in common—we animals require many of the same substances plants do. And in the same forms. So when we eat the vegetable, the fruit, the berry, the bean, the grain, the nut—the thing itself—then we get its nutrients intact and available for absorption by another living being: us. A fruit or vegetable is like the go-between—a way for us to absorb the substances that exist in the soil, in the world.

That's the amazing journey of nutrition, from the soil to the plant's cells to ours. We feed our bodies, but we nourish our cells. That's the level at which we most truly exist—each of us a miraculous collection of over 70 trillion or so cells.

A lot goes on inside our cell walls. Chemicals flow in and out on tides of fluid. Energy is generated. Messages are sent and received. Substances are created and destroyed. Debris is carried away. Our cells contain our blueprints, the genetic instructions for keeping us alive and thriving. But even our genes and chromosomes respond to their environment—to the conditions we create by our choices. We have genetic dispositions, true, but how they are expressed depends to a large degree on what we put into our mouths.

There's a whole new science devoted to this very subject—epigenetics, which looks at how and why genes express themselves. Once, we believed our genes were our destiny. Now we're learning that we have more control over them than we thought. If we maintain the health of our DNA through positive lifestyle choices—food, water, habits, even thoughts—we have a chance for long, productive lives. We can also turn on gene expression that causes disease with poor choices. If the damage to our DNA becomes too great, bad things ensue. Like cancer, to name just one.

Lately scientists have devoted lots of attention to our telomeres—the tails of our chromosomes. Telomere length is connected to how much stress—nutritional and otherwise—we put on our bodies. The more stress, the shorter the telomere length, the briefer the life. Every single food choice we make matters at the cellular and even the chromosomal levels.

As amazing as our cells and chromosomes and telomeres are, they still need us to provide the proper raw materials. To fuel all those cellular functions, we have to eat what our cells need.

So what do our cells need?

They need water, which we'll discuss in "Life Force Number Two: Hydration." Oxygen, too, which is the subject of "Life Force Number Three: Oxygenation."

And they need food. Protein. Carbohydrates. Fats. Those are the so-called macronutrients—the basic requirements of life, the substances that create our bodies and fuel them. Beyond those, we need a long list of other things just as vital, like vitamins, minerals, salts, enzymes, coenzymes, antioxidants, electrolytes, micronutrients, phytonutrients, flavonoids, carotenoids, microbes, acids, on and on. It's a lot to keep track of. Science is always discovering new ones. No way we'll remember them all.

So what's the best way to give our cells what they need? You guessed it—a wide variety of whole, fresh, clean plant-based food, a lot of it raw. Let's go through that list one by one.

# Why Whole Matters

Whole—meaning simply the entire fruit, vegetable, or whatever in its natural state—should be simple for us to manage. It's not only the healthiest, it's the easiest.

T. Colin Campbell is the author of the famed China Study, a massive twenty-year research project he directed on the relationship between nutrition and health. Here's his observation about whole food:

"Every apple contains thousands of antioxidants whose names, beyond a few like vitamin C, are unfamiliar to us, and each of these powerful chemicals has the potential to play an important role in supporting our health. They impact thousands upon thousands of metabolic reactions inside the human body. But calculating the specific influence of each of these chemicals isn't nearly sufficient to explain the effect of the apple as a whole. Because almost every chemical can affect every other chemical, there is an almost infinite number of possible biological consequences."

*An almost infinite number of possible biological consequences*, and that's from just one apple. Now imagine what's going on inside our bodies if, on a typical day, we eat a lot of whole fresh vegetables, fruit, grains, beans, nuts, and seeds. We'd get all the basic nutrients required by life, of course, but also a nearly infinite number of events that increase our well-being.

And all we have to do is eat it, and maybe show our food a little respect, a little gratitude, a little love.

But mainly, we have to eat it. As is.

Let's look at the gold standard of nutritious whole food—green, funny-looking, fibrous, satisfyingly unsweet, despised by vegetable haters everywhere, righteously good for us in every way.

Broccoli is a crucifer, one of a group of vegetables with four-petaled flowers that resemble a cross—or *crux*, in Latin, hence the name. In Italy, where it originally came from, it was a good, cheap, nutritious peasant staple. Now it's everywhere. Like every plant food, broccoli contains thousands of chemical substances, many of them still unknown even to science. But we do know that broccoli is insanely healthy. If somebody developed a pill that contained every lifesaving substance in a serving of broccoli, we would all start taking it immediately, and we'd give its inventor the Nobel Prize. But it is beyond science's ability to create such a pill, and anyway we don't need one. We can eat broccoli.

What exactly is so great about broccoli? To begin with, it's an excellent source of vitamins A, C, and K, folate, and fiber, and a good source of manganese, tryptophan, potassium, magnesium, omega-3 fatty acids, iron, calcium, zinc, vitamins B and E, and the carotenoids lutein and zeaxanthin, which protect the eyes, among other things.

It even provides something it doesn't actually contain, technically speaking—a chemical called sulforaphane, a sulfur compound. This substance doesn't exist in broccoli, but when we chew it, enzymes in our saliva combine with sulforaphane's precursors contained in the vegetable, and, presto, there it is, like a magic trick. The sulforaphane then activates two hundred different genes, some of them protecting us from cancer and others preventing the disease's spread. Sulforaphane has been found to hinder the growth of breast cancer and prostate cancer cells specifically, although its benefits appear to extend to genes everywhere in the body. It kills cancer stem cells. It normalizes DNA methylation, a process that regulates gene expression. It kills an enzyme that damages cartilage. (You thought all enzymes are good? Nature doesn't work that way.)

The other cruciferous vegetables—cauliflower, kale, Brussels sprouts, cabbage—have similar protective and disease-fighting powers. If all that sounds impressive, keep in mind that the raw sprouts of the broccoli plant have between twenty and fifty times as much of the protective chemicals as the vegetable itself.

And that's not even all the benefit they bring us! The truth is, we don't know everything that's inside a simple piece of fruit or vegetable, and even the most sophisticated laboratory analysis can't explain how all the chemicals act and interact once they enter our bodies.

As Dr. Joel Fuhrman, author of *Eat to Live*, points out, a tomato contains about ten thousand phytonutrients, many of which haven't yet been identified. In other words, even a common tomato is a mysterious force of health and healing. We can hold it, we can buy it, we can eat it, but we can't really know it.

Now, if a single vegetable contains such amazing, abundant treasure, what is the beneficial content of an entire big, varied salad? And keep in mind, sheer number of nutrients is only the beginning of the story. What matters most is how their cells react with our cells, which produce enzymes and other substances of their own, and how the chemicals and single-celled organisms in all the vegetables and spices and herbs interact—how they amplify and support and enable each other. Now add in the water we drink, the air we breathe, the energy of the sunlight we absorb. The possibilities for good things from whole food suddenly become unimaginably huge.

We will never know everything about nature's power, but we can easily harness it—by eating it whole.

Every time we try to separate one part of a food from the rest, we risk losing something important. We think we can improve upon food as nature made it, but sometimes we just screw it up. Every time we process something or pull one component out, we create an unknown. We subject our bodies to nutritional instability and the potential for chaos. That's why whole matters.

It happens when food manufacturers strip the bran from grains in order to make cereal and bread that contains no beneficial fiber or nutrients—just simple carbs, like a pure hit of sugar. Or when we squeeze the juice from fruit, discarding the pulp. Or when we extract the oil from nuts, seeds, and vegetables, essentially juicing them—using the calorie-dense fat and leaving behind the fiber.

We talk about fiber as though it is just one part of the fruit or vegetable, but truly it *is* the fruit or vegetable—the flesh itself, which contains the juice along with the nutrients and everything else. Fiber isn't just this useful stuff we need to slow down digestion and scrub our colons (though it is that, too). We don't digest fiber, but the healthy microbes in our intestines do, producing even more beneficial, protective chemicals.

Here's how dramatically food can change when we tamper with it. A large-scale study published in the *British Medical Journal* found that people who ate fruit at least twice a week—especially apples, blueberries, and grapes—were up to 23 percent less likely to develop type 2 diabetes than those who ate fruit no more than once a month. But subjects who drank fruit juice once a day or more had an *increased* risk of developing diabetes, up to 21 percent higher than those who did not.

"Our data further endorse current recommendations on increasing whole fruits, but not fruit juice, as a measure for diabetes prevention," said lead study author Isao Muraki, a research fellow with the Harvard School of Public Health's Department of Nutrition.

A study done at Pomona College and published in *Food & Nutrition Research* fed two groups of subjects meals that were identical in calories, fats, proteins, and carbs. The only difference was that one group ate all whole foods, while the other had everything processed and packaged. Then the researchers measured the calories each group metabolized—and found that those who ate processed foods burned off only half as many calories as the others. According to the authors, "this would indicate that diets with a high proportion of PFs (processed foods) will result in increased energy assimilation and may be a contributor to weight gain."

Another study, performed at Memorial University of Newfoundland, St. John's, Canada, measured how processing affects the nutraceutical content of food—the beneficial substances that act as natural medicines. "In most cases," according to the study, "processing negatively affects the bioactive components of functional foods and nutraceuticals. Therefore, minimally processed products better serve the health conscious consumers."

If the things we eat have been processed—manipulated, broken apart, adulterated, with most of the fiber (and nutrients) thrown away—then we end up consuming something that's food, technically speaking, but lacks many of the health benefits that eating is supposed to bring us. We get calories—which we need to survive, of course—but little else. None of the nutrition. As Dr. Fuhrman puts it, we end up mechanically full but nutritionally starved. If we do that often enough, we will absolutely harm ourselves at the cellular level. Over time, that may bring about some chronic condition.

Even when the calorie count is identical to what's in whole foods, as we saw in that study I quoted earlier, our metabolisms respond to processed food differently, which is really how people end up obese and unhealthy—not only because they eat too much, but because they eat too much nonwhole food.

Processed, packaged foods invariably contain things we know are bad for our cells—sugar, high-fructose corn syrup, refined wheat flour, chemical preservatives, flavorings, and coloring agents. You can read the list of ingredients and still not know everything that's in there. (Don't ask about the legal allowances for insect parts and rodent feces.) The commercial food industry has spun totally out of control—we no longer know what we're eating when we eat processed food.

But if we eat enough whole food, we won't have room left for the other kind.

# What Fresh Means

*Fresh* is one of the most overused terms when it comes to our foods. It is a word that has been co-opted by advertising and marketers to mean virtually anything. The best definition of fresh food is produce that hasn't been lying around too long before we eat it. Within hours of picking, all the protective nutrients contained in fruit or vegetables begin to break down. The light energy the plant has absorbed from the sun begins to dim.

In a 2003 study conducted by the Laboratorio de Fitoquimica, Departamento de Ciencia y Tecnología de los Alimentos, Spain, the vitamin C and flavonoid content of freshly harvested broccoli were measured, and then the vegetable was wrapped in plastic film and stored for a week at just above freezing, to simulate conditions during commercial transport and distribution. At that point the nutrients were measured again, and then once more three days later, at the end of their typical on-sale period.

According to the paper, published in the *Journal of Agricultural and Food Chemistry*, "Results showed major losses at the end of both periods, in comparison with broccoli at harvest. Thus, the respective losses, at the end of cold storage and retail periods, were 71 and 80 percent of total glucosinolates [cancer-fighting chemicals], 62 and 51 percent of total flavonoids, 44 and 51 percent of sinapic acid derivatives, and 73 and 74 percent of caffeoyl-quinic acid derivatives. Slight differences in all compound concentrations between storage and retail sale periods were detected."

In short, that ten-day period killed off significant amounts of the good things that broccoli contained at the moment it was picked. "Distribution and retail periods had minimal effects on vitamin C," according to the paper, but that's not much comfort.

The word *fresh*, when speaking about produce, also means that it has been allowed to grow until it is fully mature, or ripe—when all its nutrients and enzymes are at their peak—before it is picked. This is just as crucial.

When the fruit is immature, so are all its contents. Vitamins, minerals, enzymes, and antioxidants need time to fully develop. If we pick produce when it is underripe, we unplug it prematurely from its source of nutrition, the soil, thereby depriving it (and us) of potential benefit. By the time we eat it, the produce may look beautiful and ripe and nutritious. But because it was picked when immature, the nutrients just aren't there.

Researchers from the Department of Pomology, University of California–Davis, in a paper titled "Preharvest and Postharvest Factors Influencing Vitamin C Content of Horticultural Crops," measured how various factors, among them the maturity of the fruits and vegetables at the time of picking, affect vitamin C content of produce. "While full color may be achieved after harvest," the authors wrote, "nutritional quality may not. Total vitamin C content of red peppers, tomatoes, apricots, peaches and papayas has been shown to be higher when these crops are picked ripe from the plant."

Of course, that eliminates virtually everything we buy in stores and supermarkets, since all produce that is shipped any distance has to be picked before it is ripe, or it will be mush by the time we get it.

What's the solution? First, we need to eat all the plant-based foods we can, to make up for any lack of nutrients in them. But we also need to do everything we can to get our fruit and vegetables as fresh as possible, with the shortest amount of time from harvest to table.

We do that, first, by paying attention to the produce we buy, especially its place of origin. Once upon a time fruits and vegetables were seasonal—they were available at certain times of the year and not others. Transportation and refrigeration brought an end to that quaint idea, and now we can find anything at just about any time. There are no seasons now, where most produce is concerned. We may see that as progress, but it's a mixed blessing at best.

An apple grown ten miles away and an apple grown fifteen hundred miles away are not equal, even though we seem to be comparing apples and apples. Should we eat a Fuji apple from New Zealand or a melon apple from Minnesota? That's a no-brainer even if you prefer the Fuji variety. Better to go without something for a few months than to eat it when it's out of season on our continent.

Actually, frozen fruits and vegetables, especially if organic, are preferable to unfrozen produce that has traveled great distances. Fresh conventionally grown blueberries from Argentina or frozen organic wild blueberries from Canada? I choose the latter. I'm a fanatic about fresh, but most of the year I eat frozen berries. A ripe fruit that's frozen as soon as it's picked will retain nutrients that a fresh fruit picked unripe will never possess.

Another strategy is to get as much food as possible from a farm stand or farmers' market. The locavore argument isn't just philosophical—it makes a genuine difference in the level of nutrition if we eat things that were grown close to home and picked recently. Buying from small farmers also keeps some of the food supply out of the hands of the agribusiness giants. That's good for our health, too. The small growers actually touch (and eat) the things they grow.

Starting an organic garden is a great way to get fresh food. Grow it at home or nearby without chemicals, pick it at its peak, eat it five minutes later (if not right off the stem). Even a single tree or the smallest patch of dirt can yield a lot of produce and herbs, enough to make a genuine difference in our well-being. And it reconnects us with our food—we're bound to take more care preparing and eating something we've raised ourselves. Growing our own food is a great way of taking more responsibility for our health.

A final way to make sure we're getting fresh vegetables is to eat the sprout instead of the vegetable itself. As we said before, the sprout almost always has a much higher nutrient content than the full-grown produce.

A study of cereal grains that were allowed to sprout before they were eaten was conducted at the Department of Biochemistry at Mahatma Phule Agricultural University, India, and published in *Critical Reviews in Food Science and Nutrition*. "Sprouting of grains for a limited period," the researchers concluded, "causes increased activities of hydrolytic enzymes, improvement in the contents of certain essential amino acids, total sugars, and B-group vitamins, and a decrease in dry matter, starch, and antinutrients."

In another study, German researchers sprouted wheat kernels for up to a week, analyzing them at different stages to learn the effects of germination on nutrients. Overall, the sprouting process decreased gluten proteins substantially while increasing folate, a win-win. According to a paper published in the *Journal of Agriculture and Food Chemistry*, longer germination times "led to a substantial increase of total dietary fiber and to a strong increase of the soluble dietary fiber," with soluble fiber tripling and insoluble fiber decreasing by half.

You can find a variety of sprouts in most health food stores. They're really easy to grow at home, too. You need some organic seeds, a little water, jars or growing trays, and sunlight. Before you know it, you will have the most intensely nutritious food in the world, year-round and cheap.

As our food supply has been transformed by industrialization, the question of freshness has become much more urgent. Once, even city dwellers lived near the farms that grew our food. No longer. Now it comes from all over the planet. Do we really think that this change has no effect on food's quality, or on our ability to know or control what we're eating? Do we have any idea of the conditions under which it was grown and picked and handled? No. Do we know anything about the quality of the soil and air and water where it grew? No. And all these factors are important—these are the things that nourished our food before it arrived on our kitchen tables to nourish us.

A study published in 1997 in the *British Food Journal* looked at how nutrient levels in produce had declined over a fifty-year period. The average content of calcium in vegetables had declined to 81 percent of its original level. There were significant reductions in the levels of magnesium, copper, and sodium in vegetables and magnesium, iron, copper, and potassium in fruits. The greatest change was the reduction of copper content in vegetables, to less than one-fifth of the old level. The only mineral that showed no significant difference over the fifty-year period was phosphorus. Also, "Water increased significantly and dry matter decreased significantly in fruits," according to the study, meaning the food contained less fiber, and so less nutrition and flavor, than before.

Scientists from the Bio-Communications Research Institute and the Biochemical Institute of the University of Texas tracked nutrient changes in forty-three garden crops from 1950 to 1999. "As a group," the report said, "the 43 foods show apparent, statistically reliable declines for 6 nutrients (protein, calcium, phosphorus, iron, riboflavin and ascorbic acid)."

The lead researcher, Dr. Donald R. Davis, said, "We conclude that the most likely explanation was changes in cultivated varieties used today compared to 50 years ago. During those 50 years, there have been intensive efforts to breed new varieties that have greater yield, or resistance to pests, or adaptability to different climates. But the dominant effort is for higher yields. Emerging evidence suggests that when you select for yield, crops grow bigger and faster, but they don't necessarily have the ability to make or uptake nutrients at the same, faster rate."

## Why Variety Is So Important

Once, scientists tell us, before agriculture, humans ate hundreds of varieties of fruit and vegetables, all wild, each a little different from the others. Today, the average diet contains around thirty foods. What kind of difference do you think that makes to our health?

"Evolutionarily, our bodies were designed to eat a variety of foods," says Emory University anthropologist George Armelagos. "Our hunter and gatherer ancestors ate a wide selection of whole foods often, to escape food boredom. Today, although it appears our food system offers a wide variety of ingredients, in reality, our diets are primarily composed of foods high in corn products and refined sugar."

According to Dr. Michael Greger, the physician behind the

website nutritionfacts.org, prehistoric man probably took in around 10,000 mg of potassium a day, all from vegetables and fruit. Today, according to US government figures, fewer than 2 percent of us get the recommended daily minimum of less than half that, 4,700 mg. And that's just one nutrient, although potassium is a pretty important one, especially where cardiovascular health is concerned. According to a study published in the *Journal of the American College of Cardiology*, a 1,600 mg increase in daily potassium consumption led to a 21 percent lower risk of stroke.

Dr. Carolyn Dean, medical director of the Nutritional Magnesium Association, says that a deficiency of that important mineral has also become common. Dietary levels of magnesium from both food and water have gradually declined in the United States, she reports, from a high of 500 mg a day in 1900 to barely 175–225 mg a day today. The National Academy of Sciences has found that most American men consume only about 80 percent of the recommended daily allowance (RDA) of magnesium, and women only 70 percent.

Even similar foods can have significantly different nutritional profiles. Kale and broccoli are both cruciferous vegetables, both extremely healthy. But according to the USDA database, a cup of raw kale has 100 mg of calcium and 329 mg of potassium, with a total of 33 calories. A cup of raw broccoli has only 43 mg of calcium and 288 of potassium, with 31 calories. But that doesn't mean we should give up broccoli in favor of kale, because—as we've seen—broccoli has a great many other beneficial substances. So: eat broccoli *and* kale.

That's why eating a variety of foods is so important. As we've noted, even scientists can't list every nutrient contained in the plant foods we eat. But we know that they all contribute to our health. The less varied our diet, the fewer nutrients we get. It's that simple.

In a paper titled "Food Variety as a Quantitative Descriptor of Food Intake," Professor Mark L. Wahlqvist, who served as president of the International Union of Nutritional Science, wrote,

"The major reason for inclusion of food variety as a dietary guideline is the generally accepted concept that eating a wider variety of foods improves nutrient adequacy."

We go to the store to buy cabbage, not realizing there are literally hundreds of different varieties in existence, each slightly different, with its own signature nutrients. In a perfect world, we'd eat them all.

Of course, there's a practical obstacle to getting more variety in our food. Demanding it would require our neighborhood supermarket to carry a dozen different kinds of cabbage, and our agricultural giants would have to grow and market all those varieties, and that wouldn't be easy. That's the real reason we're forced to live in a kind of vegetal poverty: the profit motive.

So we need to look harder. We have to seek out new kinds of kale, lettuce, tomato, squash, herbs, even if we love the old ones. Be promiscuous about it. Don't be so faithful to the old standbys that you won't try a new taste. Get into your food a little more, enough to tell the difference between one kind of onion and another. Put your face right in there and inhale. We don't use our olfactory sense enough. Ripe plants have such a strong, seductive perfume—the desire they create is almost sexual, sensual indeed, like the scent of a lover's body. It actually is sexual. In the wild, that aroma is one way plants get the attention of the birds and the bees.

The modern produce industry has given us food that doesn't smell much like anything. Often it doesn't taste like much either. No wonder we don't get excited by the prospect of a new variety of pear or pepper—we can't really tell the difference. A pepper is a pepper—no! Not any more than all sex is the same.

This is how well the junk food giants understand the physiology of hunger: Open a bag of Doritos and take a whiff of the overpowering perfume of fat, salt, and sugar. It's a carefully manufactured scent and taste sensation meant to trick you into thinking you are eating something essential. We're being manipulated by food engineers who have figured out how to tap into our brains. But if we can kick our addiction to junk food, we become better able to distinguish the fake stuff from the real, and that chemical aroma will lose its power to hook us.

The question of nutrient diversity is a good reason for going crazy with salads. They tend to contain a mix of raw, whole plant foods untainted by anything else. That's what a big chunk of our food intake should resemble: one big, daylong salad menu, course after course of fresh, whole vegetables, sprouts, fruits, beans, nuts, and seeds. Dressing, of course, made with a healthy fat such as olive, sesame, walnut, or avocado oil, or the somewhat exotic but very beneficial oil from the sacha inchi seed. All cold-pressed, and without the bad bottled dressing, cheese, meat, croutons, bacon bits, or other add-ons that contribute cheap carbs, unhealthy fats, and unnecessary calories. Want that salad sweeter to balance out the bitter greens? Throw in some fresh fruit, or a handful of raisins, dried cranberries, or dried cherries. Need a little bulk in there? Add a big scoop of hummus, a cut-up avocado, or a fistful of walnuts. Some healthy protein? Soak raw quinoa in warm water for half an hour to soften it, then sprinkle it on top, or add some black beans.

Clearly, we're no longer talking about a dainty little bowl with some lettuce, tomato, and cucumber, maybe some shaved carrots for color, and a splash of dressing. Today, salad has to be epic—a meal, not a course. We need bigger bowls.

Every salad I make is a little different from all the others. I never put the same things into two smoothies, either. If variety really is the spice of life, then the lack of it equals tasteless meals.

There's another good reason for eating a diverse diet. Each fruit and vegetable contains toxins along with the nutrients. The irritants and repellents are there to fend off herbivores who might otherwise overfeed. Some substances act as natural pesticides, and there are even insect contraceptives contained in some plants. If we vary our produce, we won't get too much of any one harmful thing. But if we keep eating the same plants over and over, their toxins or enzyme inhibitors may build up and eventually cause allergic reactions or even hurt us.

## Clean Means Natural

When we're talking about food, clean doesn't mean "not dirty"—in fact, dirt is probably the cleanest thing our food comes into contact with. Clean means free of harmful chemical pesticides, larvacides, herbicides, and fertilizers. Clean means organic or wild harvested.

People sometimes ask me, "Why should I spend more money for organic when the vegetables are the same?" Well, that's the whole point: they're *not* the same.

Pesticides and herbicides kill—that's their job. They eliminate insects that eat plants and destroy crops, and control nuisance weeds and other plants. But if something can kill a bug, do we really think it's going to be healthy for us?

In 2004 researchers from the National Institutes of Health published a study that found an increased cancer risk among 17,000 children living on farms where pesticide use had also increased. Studies have linked exposure to organophosphate and organochlorines (chemicals commonly found in pesticides) to several kinds of cancer, leukemia, lymphoma, Parkinson's disease, ALS, fetal birth defects, asthma and other respiratory ailments, ADHD, diabetes, and even increased risk of death due to heart disease.

And the deadly chemicals used in farming don't go away just because they've been outlawed. An article published in the journal *Neurotoxicology* noted that even though the pesticide dieldrin has been banned, it continues to exist in the environment, and has been found in Parkinson's disease sufferers' postmortem brain tissues.

We can wash off some pesticides with water, vinegar, or hydrogen peroxide. But that doesn't take care of the threat entirely. The problem isn't only the pesticides. It's that the pesticides will join all the other industrial toxins—the harmful food additives, environmental pollution, and everyday chemical irritants we come into contact with, now, in the past, and in the future. At some point our immune systems just become overwhelmed. When that happens, something may slip through our defenses. A disease-causing bacterium or virus will find a hospitable place to grow. A carcinogen will take root and begin to spread.

All these chemicals keep adding up, meal by meal, day by day, year by year. That's the real danger—accumulation. The government can assure us that exposure to a particular pesticide below a certain level has been proven harmless. But how do the government rule makers know what else we're being exposed to? Obviously, they don't. And believe me, there's more than one straw on this camel's back.

That's why we have a million rules, and yet we keep getting sick and dying from cancer and Parkinson's disease. The rules exist to tell companies what they can get away with, not to protect us.

A study performed at Stanford University got a lot of attention for claiming that there's no meaningful difference in nutrient content between organic and nonorganic produce. A lot of people want to believe that, for obvious reasons. But even that study found higher levels of vitamin C in organic strawberries. The organic produce it measured also contained more phenols, plant compounds believed to help prevent cancer, than conventional produce. And other research has found organic foods to be healthier than those grown using pesticides.

Researchers at Washington State University's Center for Sustaining Agriculture and Natural Resources looked at 384 samples of organic and conventional milk taken over eighteen months around the country. The organic milk contained 62 percent more omega-3 fatty acids (which we tend to need more of) and 25 percent less omega-6s (which we tend to have in excess). This doesn't mean that drinking cow's milk is healthy—it isn't, especially for adults. But it shows there can be nutritional benefits to eating organic.

A study published in *Chemistry Central Journal* measured carotenoids, total polyphenols, and antioxidant activity in the skins of wine and table grapes grown both organically and conventionally. The organic grapes had significantly more of all the beneficial substances. Another study, done by the Department of Food Science and Technology of the University of California–Davis, compared content of phenolic—a measure of antioxidant activity—and ascorbic acid (vitamin C) in strawberries, marionberries, and corn grown conventionally and organically. According to the report, "Statistically higher levels of TP (Total Phenolic) were consistently found in organically and sustainably grown foods as compared to those produced by conventional agricultural practices."

In 2001 the *Journal of Alternative and Complementary Medicine* published an article on the nutritional value of organic versus conventional plant-based foods. "Organic crops contained significantly more Vitamin C, iron, magnesium and phosphorus and significantly less nitrates than conventional crops," it said. "There appear to be genuine differences in the nutrient content of organic and conventional crops."

One thing we know for sure: no scientist has ever shown that pesticides are good for us.

Eating organic absolutely means we're lessening our toxic load, which is kind to the liver and kidneys, which have enough to do these days. Eating organic lowers stress on the entire body, not just the digestive system. There are new agricultural chemicals being developed all the time. Nobody can say for sure what the long-term effects will be for each and every one.

It's true, organic food is more expensive to grow, and we have to be willing to pay for it. Some people see that as a luxury. I always come back to the same question: Would we rather give our money to the farmer or the pharmacist, the grocer or the doctor? Do we want to spend a fortune in the future trying to fix the damage being done today? Once we compare the potential risk and reward, the extra cost of eating clean food may seem worth it. Eating is the single most important thing we can do to stay healthy. If good, clean food isn't worth our money, what is?

Organic blackberries cost double the normal kind? How does that compare to the price of chemotherapy? How does burning out your insides with toxic chemicals and destroying your immune system and puking out your guts and losing all your hair stack up against spending three dollars more on that organic produce?

Your body responds to what you put inside it. It's simple. How could anything else be possible? You'd accept that if we were talking about your car. Why not your body?

Clean also means food that contains no genetically modified organisms—GMOs. This is the really scary stuff, and it's in the news every day as the big corporations fight every effort to label engineered foods. The fact that the industry is against truth in labeling tells us all we need to know.

GMOs are seeds and grains that have been altered at the DNA level. Their genes have been manipulated, usually to make them pest-resistant. What exactly is the harm of humans eating food containing GMOs? That's the point—we don't know. They haven't been around long enough to determine the long-term effects. That's a good reason to avoid them, in my book. It shouldn't be our responsibility to prove GMOs are unsafe—the companies that develop and sell them should have to run tests demonstrating that they pose no threat to our health. I don't want to be an unpaid lab rat for Monsanto, do you? I will put my trust in nature, not a chemical company driven by profit.

In 2012 researchers from the University of Caen, France, published the results of a two-year study of rats fed a diet consisting of a Monsanto genetically modified corn compared to rats fed non-GMO corn. The ones exposed to the GMOs, they reported, died sooner than the control group and had higher rates of tumors and organ damage. A few months later the American scientific journal that published the study retracted it, supposedly because it was too inconclusive. But some scientists criticized that decision as politically motivated. One called it "scientific censorship."

Maybe someday, people say, the technology of GMOs will be used for good and be proven healthy. Good luck with that, I say. I'll continue to eat as naturally and cleanly as I can.

# Why Raw Matters

There are lots of good reasons for eating food raw.

First, raw food retains all its water, which improves our hydration. Raw food also alkalizes our tissues, while cooking it can make us more acidic, which can lead to problems (we'll discuss this in "Life Force Number Four: Alkalization").

All those benefits we discussed that come from the sulforaphane contained in broccoli? We get them as long as the vegetable hasn't been cooked at very high temperatures. The heat kills certain nutrients. So whether we eat broccoli itself or the sprouts, we need to get at least some of it raw.

Of course, not many of us would be happy following a strictly raw food diet. I've done it, and it works for me only for short periods of time. It's a pretty radical way to go. Cooking is an important part of what makes us human, and it makes eating a lot tastier, not to mention more interesting and diverse. Still, it's worthwhile to note the health effects of an all-raw diet.

In one study, done at the University of Kuopio, Finland, and published in the *American Journal of Clinical Nutrition*, the antioxidant levels of middle-aged Finnish vegans living on a 100 percent raw food diet were compared to the levels found in Finns eating omnivorously. Compared to the omnivores, the vegans had significantly higher blood concentrations of beta-carotene, vitamin C, and vitamin E, as well as greater overall antioxidant activity.

In fact, based on USDA recommended dietary allowances, the vegans in the study were getting an amazing 305 percent of daily vitamin C requirements, 247 percent of vitamin A, 313 percent of vitamin E, 120 percent of copper, 92 percent of zinc, and 49 percent of selenium. We Americans, for the most part, don't get even the recommended amounts of these vitamins and nutrients.

Another study, done by the German Institute of Nutritional Science, found that an all-raw diet "lowers plasma total cholesterol and triglyceride concentrations," indicating good heart health.

Like I said, going all-raw isn't an appetizing option for most of us. But these studies and many others like them make it clear: the more raw plant-based food we eat, the healthier we'll be. Plain and simple.

One of the best reasons for eating uncooked vegetables and fruits is this: they hang on to all their enzymes. And enzymes are very, very important to our health. Enzymes aren't nutrients, strictly speaking. But without them we couldn't make use of any of the nutrients we eat.

Made of chains of protein molecules, enzymes act as catalysts for every single biochemical event that happens inside us. Not just in our digestive systems, either—everywhere. There are thousands of different enzymes, and each does just one specific thing. We need them all.

It's hard to exaggerate the importance of enzymes to the functioning human body. Imagine if you were building a road and you made sure to have all the materials and machinery in place to start construction, but you forgot to hire any workers. That's our bodies if we didn't have enzymes. No road.

Digestive enzymes help break down food into components that can be absorbed, transported, and utilized by every cell in our bodies. Without enough of these, we won't fully benefit from the nutrients we eat.

Systemic enzymes are involved in everything else that happens in our bodies—they help regulate our circulatory, lymphatic, cardiac, neurological, endocrine, renal, hepatic, and reproductive systems. They also maintain our skin, bones, joints, muscles, and other tissues, and they cleanse our blood and help fight inflammation.

Enzymatic activity is complex. A digestive enzyme will turn a nutrient into an acid, and then another enzyme turns that acid into a different acid, and this may happen repeatedly, step after step, until at last the result is a substance the body can use.

Our bodies systemic create enzymes in the liver and pancreas, but our livers have a lot else to do these days, neutralizing all the toxins we take in. We need to cut that overworked organ a break when we can, which is why it's so important that we get enzymes from external sources, meaning foods and enzyme supplements.

There are eight main enzymes that allow us to access the nutrients in food. One is specifically meant for protein (protease); others break down dairy (lactase), fiber (cellulase), fats (lipase), and so on. They are positioned wherever our bodies need them to be. For instance, the enzyme that breaks down carbs, amylase, is present in our saliva, which starts the digestive process inside our mouths as we chew.

Most whole foods contain the enzyme that helps break them down. It's a neat little self-contained system. Milk, for example, contains the enzyme lactase, which helps digest the lactose that is also present.

Once milk is pasteurized, though—heated to a temperature high enough to kill potentially harmful microbes—the enzymes are killed too. Without that lactase, lactose is difficult for our bodies to handle, which is why so many people can't tolerate it.

That's the main problem we face when it comes to enzymes in our diet. They begin to die soon after vegetables or fruit are picked, and heating food to over 118 degrees Fahrenheit kills them, meaning the enzymes are already dead by the time we eat most things, even healthy ones. Processed foods, by definition, are devoid of usable digestive enzymes.

A lack of enzymatic action causes incomplete digestion of the foods we eat. We don't extract from them all the nutrition they contain, and what we don't take, we still need to metabolize and excrete. Those wastes will be in the form of acids, which raise the overall acidity level of our bodies. Excess acidity also damages our ability to produce more enzymes. As a result, digestion worsens and acidic wastes increase. This becomes an unhealthy cascade of events—improper eating makes us acidic, which damages our enzymes, which makes us more acidic. You will read about adverse effects of acidity later in this book.

Poor enzymatic action is also blamed for a number of physical ailments, from degenerative diseases to poor aging to chronic inflammation and pain.

In a study published in *Cancer Chemotherapy and Pharmacology*, patients who had undergone surgery and treatment for colorectal cancer were also given digestive enzymes. The enzyme therapy improved the quality of the subjects' lives "by reducing both the signs and symptoms of the disease."

It's clear—we need to eat whole foods, and eat a significant portion of them raw, so the enzymes are still alive and active. This is why it's so important to eat big salads with lots of uncooked vegetables, not just lettuce. We need the enzymes.

In the back of this book I list foods that are rich in enzymes. Some good examples are pineapple, papaya, avocado, raw honey, and bee pollen. Meat actually contains a lot of enzymes. Of course, once it's cooked, they die. If we limited ourselves to steak tartare, we might be all right—if the *E. coli* didn't get us, that is. But digesting meat requires quite a lot of enzymes, meaning it becomes a severe strain on enzymatic action. Next thing you know, the meat is lying around in our stomachs, putrefying—*rotting*—and creating a buildup of toxins and bad bacteria.

Keep in mind, some veggies actually become healthier when cooked. Tomatoes, when heated, release lycopene, a potent cancer fighter. Carrots, spinach, asparagus, and some mushrooms produce more carotenoids and ferulic acid, both antioxidants, when lightly steamed or slow-cooked. But even that comes at a cost— they also lose some of their water-soluble nutrients, like vitamin

C. So, again, diversity in food is a good thing, and cooking can also be a benefit to health.

# Every Bite Counts

It's all very simple!

We need to focus on saying yes to good, healthy foods rather than concentrating on the things we shouldn't eat. (In "Nutritional Stress," we'll discuss the dangers in giving our cells the things they don't need.) But if we eat right, everything else takes care of itself. That's one of the advantages to eating as I've described in this chapter: we need a lot of good quality food to keep ourselves properly nourished. That should come as good news to those of us who are constantly worrying about eating too much.

The other important lesson is that we need to pay attention to everything we eat. We have to reconnect with our food and really know what's in each meal. There's no other way to be sure we're getting what we need. That's another reason that fresh, clean whole foods are the right way to go—there's never a question about what's in them.

We need to remember that every bite we take is a decision: healthy or unhealthy? Will this food nourish me, will it deliver something needed to my cells, will it enhance my well-being? Maybe the answer won't always be yes. It's hard to live up to any ideal. But what happens if we make more good decisions than bad ones? When we eat right, we benefit ourselves not just today and tomorrow but twenty, thirty, fifty years from now.

When we eat poorly, the opposite is true—we do harm in the here and now but also perpetuate conditions that may be deadly in the future. We won't be able to go back and uneat that fast-food pig-out or add a daily big green salad and vegetables to the diet of our past. Though we may wish we could.

# Simple To-Do List ✓

- Aim for a daily diet made up mostly of fresh, whole vegetables, fruit, beans, nuts, seeds and healthy fats. Meat should be an occasional meal at most, and from creatures that are organically grown and humanely raised; fish should be wild-caught.

- Whole food, not pills, should be the primary source of our most important nutrients—minerals such as calcium, magnesium, potassium, sodium, sulfur, and all our vitamins.

- Eat at least one meal a day of raw vegetables or fruit (or both). It's why salads and smoothies are so important to a healthy diet.

- Food grown organically and close to home is the absolute best thing we can eat. That's as near to nutritional perfection as we're ever going to get.

- Variety isn't just the spice of life, it also ensures that we get all the different micronutrients we need. Every time you see a new type of fruit, vegetable, or bean, give it a chance.

- Eat more sprouts. They're a lot easier to grow at home and are a source of powerful goodness.

- Let your senses be your guide—eat real food that is beautiful and smells good!

# Feeding Our Other Body

As we've already said, we have lots of human cells to feed and care for, around 70-plus trillion of them. But that's hardly all of it—we also need to nourish about ten times as many nonhuman cells that our bodies contain. These are our microbes, the single-celled organisms—bacteria, viruses, fungi, yeasts—that exist inside us and on the surface of our bodies. They are not *us*, technically speaking, but they are vitally important to our health and completely necessary to our existence. Think of microbes as our roommates.

And like us, they need to eat too.

We acquired them at birth from our mothers, and they will continue to thrive inside us after we're dead. They may not even notice the difference. After we're gone they'll really live it up, feasting on us until there's nothing tasty left, at which point they will move on. We are in a cycle of life, and they are a major part of it.

Microbes have gotten a lot of bad press, which has convinced some of us that they all need to be killed off. Clever marketing has made Purell a household name. We take antibiotics at the first hint of a cough. But microbes constitute 80 percent of our immune system. Beneficial bacteria keep the harmful ones in check. When we resort to miracle drugs, we wipe out good microbes along with the bad. We've made antibiotics such a staple of modern life that bacteria have learned to adapt, meaning they've become resistant to drugs. If we're not careful, we'll be back where we were before antibiotics existed—vulnerable to every bad microbe that comes along.

Some microbes *do* cause disease, of course. We call them germs or pathogens, but those are just labels. If the conditions inside our bodies aren't hospitable to specific microbes, they don't last long enough to make us ill. As we discuss in "Life Force Number Five: Detoxification," our challenge is to create an internal environment that's inhospitable to disease-causing bacteria and viruses. We do this by eating and drinking and living in a way that supports our overall health as well as our immune systems.

Some microbes, on the other hand, are helpful. We have hundreds of species of good bacteria on our skin, for example, and they protect us by eating bad bacteria before they can penetrate our defenses. So go easy with the Purell. You're killing the good bugs, too.

By far the most plentiful and important microbes we carry are those in our gut—our intestines. These bacteria perform an important function: they help break down the foods we eat. They are absolutely necessary—they allow us to gain access to nutrients. But the microbes don't do it because they love us and want us to be healthy. It's how they survive, too.

An estimated five hundred different species of microbes live in our gut, each with a distinct and specific function and nutritional needs. Some microbes have evolved alongside human hosts to consume certain substances, such as nondigestible fiber. Others consume proteins. Still others prefer carbohydrates and sugars. Our gut flora makeup is directly influenced by the dietary choices we make. We decide which microbes to feed and which to starve. We create the ecosystem for them.

A study published in the journal *Nature* fed one group of human subjects an animal-based diet and another a plant diet. Then researchers studied the short-term results in the subjects' gut microbes. Even after just a few days, the meat eaters experienced an increase in bacteria that cause inflammatory bowel disease. The plant eaters increased the number of microbes that rid the body of inflammation. "These results demonstrate that the gut microbiome can rapidly respond to altered diet," the authors wrote.

Our microbes don't just sit around waiting for us to eat the things they need. They are capable of sending out signals, actual cravings for specific kinds of food. Then we get the sudden urge for a sweet snack, and we think it's a lack of willpower that makes us give in. Microbes also send messages telling us whether we're full. We think it's our own bodies, our own metabolisms, talking to us. But we could be wrong. There's a reason microbes have been around almost as long as the planet itself. They know how to get their way.

If we feed ourselves sugary, processed foods, then the microbes that thrive on them will proliferate and dominate our digestive system. And we will suffer. If we eat healthy foods, then the microbes that consume them will flourish. And so will we. That is a healthy symbiosis between us and them.

Pretty amazing, right? It's like a horror movie in there—we've been colonized by foreign beings telling us to do things we might not do otherwise. And we obey, thinking *we're* the ones who want that ice cream, without ever knowing that we're being played. You've heard people say, "Well, my gut tells me . . ." They weren't kidding. Our gut really does talk to us.

Scientists still have much to learn about microbes and how they operate in the human body, but we already know that they are an extremely powerful force in our lives and our health. Taken all together, they form something like their own internal organ. Scientists have begun referring to our microbiome—the term for the entire microbial being we each contain—as "the second brain." And like any other organ, it can be healthy or sick.

The microbe population inside each of us is as distinctive as a fingerprint. It's partly a matter of heredity, but mainly it's about which microbes we consume and encourage, and which ones we don't. What we eat and drink is what makes the difference. We can't fight our microbes. We have to make them work for us, not against us.

Consuming a diverse, high-fiber plant-based diet that includes fermented foods such as kimchi or sauerkraut creates a healthy intestinal environment that improves digestion, nutritional uptake, elimination, immunity, and disease prevention. Today lots of people take prebiotic supplements, which feed the "friendly" bacteria, and probiotics, which are the actual bacteria. But if we eat healthy, diverse diets, we can get all the prebiotics and bacteria we need from our food.

Most of our gut microbes exist in the lower intestine. Because processed foods are so lacking in fiber and nutrients, they are digested long before they get that far down. To sustain sufficient quantities of the healthiest bacteria, therefore, we need to eat a lot of raw and cooked whole vegetables and fruit. Foods high in fiber will reach our lower intestines relatively intact, ferment there amid all those microbes, and keep our microbiome populous and lively.

We don't digest the fiber that we eat, but a lot of our beneficial bacteria do, and they turn it into chemicals that promote our good health. One such by-product, propionate, inhibits the synthesis of cholesterol and fights obesity. Intestinal bacteria that digest fiber also produce a short-chain fatty acid called butyrate, which boosts the immune system, decreases inflammation, and protects us from cancer. In a recent study Japanese researchers found that butyrate lessened colon inflammation in lab mice. "These findings could be applicable for the prevention and treatment of inflammatory bowel disease, allergy and autoimmune disease," said Dr. Hiroshi Ohno, who led the team of scientists. "Butyrate is natural and safe as a therapy, and in addition it is cheap, which could reduce costs for both patients and society."

Many of us—a quarter of all subjects, in a study done at the University of Copenhagen—lack sufficient bacteria in the gut, as well as lacking diversity in the bacteria present. These conditions have been linked to obesity as well as chronic inflammation of the intestine.

Leaky gut syndrome—a condition in which some of the bacteria, toxins, and wastes that are supposed to remain inside the intestines escape into the bloodstream—has gotten a lot of attention over the past few years. When it was first noticed, some medical experts doubted its existence. There are fewer doubters today.

In "The Protein-Fat Myths," we'll discuss the fact that shortly after we eat animal products, our blood becomes inflamed, reacting as though foreign invaders are present. Researchers believe that this is because bacteria contained in the meat escape our digestive tract and enter the body itself, and may be the result of an unhealthy microbiome.

When food containing fiber reaches the lower intestine and ferments there, it produces short-chain fatty acids. They're important because they strengthen the cells of the intestinal walls, preventing bacteria from leaking out into our bloodstreams and causing havoc in our bodies.

Scientists are just beginning to understand all the ways our microbes influence our health. They even alter our psychological state, sending out signals that make us moody and depressed. In the past few years we've seen evidence that the gut microbiome can influence neural development, brain chemistry, pain perception, and a wide range of behaviors. Research has found, for example, that tweaking the balance between beneficial and disease-causing bacteria in an animal's gut can lead it to become either more bold or more anxious.

In a study done by the UCLA Division of Digestive Diseases and published in the journal *Gastroenterology*, thirty-six women were divided into three groups. One ate yogurt with probiotics; the second was given a yogurt-like drink containing no probiotics; and the third group was given nothing. After four weeks, the probiotic group had measurably higher brain function. The scientists concluded: "There are studies showing that what we eat can alter the composition and products of the gut flora—in particular, that people with high-vegetable, fiber-based diets have a different composition of their microbiome, or gut environment, than people who eat the more typical Western diet that is high in fat and carbohydrates. Now we know that this has an effect not only on the metabolism but also [on] brain function."

And the messaging goes both ways. The brain can also exert a powerful influence on gut bacteria; several studies have shown that even mild stress can tip the microbial balance in the gut, making the host more vulnerable to infectious disease and triggering a cascade of molecular reactions that feed back to the central nervous system. When microbial transplants were done on lab mice, the recipients' brain chemistry and even their behavior began resembling that of the donors.

Today, the study of the human microbiome is one of the most exciting fields in science. But none of this is new. Back at the turn of the twentieth century, the Russian Nobel laureate Ilya Mechnikov theorized that when certain intestinal bacteria digest proteins, they produce toxins that make our internal environment acidic and promote aging. He imagined that eating fermented dairy—he used sour milk—would introduce microbes that could decrease our intestinal acidity and promote health and longevity. Since then, probiotics have been found to have an anticarcinogenic effect and to alleviate ailments like irritable bowel, high cholesterol, and hypertension.

We've come a long way since yogurt. Lately a somewhat radical surgical form of supplementation—fecal microbiome transplantation—has been used successfully to improve the intestines' bacterial environment. A small amount of feces from a healthy person is implanted in the gut of someone suffering from an intestinal ailment. Instantly, the microbial composition changes for the better.

Yes, that's correct—poop transplants. And not only did the recipients' health improve, but they even ended up with food cravings similar to those of the donors.

I'm hoping that you won't ever need this kind of surgical intervention. But it underscores the mysterious power of our microbes over our well-being, and reminds us of the importance of caring for the nonhuman being we all carry around inside us.

# Simple To-Do List

- The bacteria we host in our gut amounts to another internal organ. Feed it properly and take care not to weaken it by eating the wrong things or exposing it to harmful industrial products.

- Sugar and processed grains encourage the proliferation of bacteria that thrive on these things, and in turn, those microbes send messages to our brain, creating urges for more unhealthy foods. Instead of relying on willpower to resist junk food, just eat better and the cravings will vanish, I promise.

- Be extremely wary of antibiotics, since these powerful drugs kill the good bacteria along with the bad. Pharmaceuticals should be the last resort, not the first. Even alcohol-based hand sanitizers and antibacterial soaps should be avoided.

- Our microbes even influence our moods and emotional state. It's worthwhile to consider changing your diet as a means to improve your outlook on life.

- Every day we should actively improve our microbiota by eating foods that contain high levels of beneficial bacteria. Sauerkraut, miso soup, yogurt, and kefir are just a few that can make a positive difference.

# Life Force Number Two:
# Hydration

I magine if we had one organ that took up two-thirds of our bodies.

It would be a huge deal, right? Its care would be a major medical specialty. There would be doctors, research institutes, universities, entire hospitals devoted to that single organ's well-being. We would forever be reading articles telling us how to maintain its optimal health. We would all know what to do to keep it running properly.

This organ doesn't really exist. But in essence, that's exactly the role water plays.

Water does make up two-thirds of our bodies. It is the universal currency of life on Earth, the unified field for all the genuine organs. Water is a major component of every kind of tissue we have, from blood to bone and everything in between. The list of jobs water does puts all those other organs to shame. And the roster of diseases and disorders that can be caused by problems with our water supply is just as impressive.

Just like any organ, our water supply can be healthy and vibrant and functioning, or it can be insufficient to do its jobs right. If we pay attention to the water we contain, and look after its health, we will instantly improve our chances for a vital, thriving life. We'll automatically begin to feel incredible benefits. Listen to me, please: everything depends on the water we drink. Acknowledging that is the single easiest way to improve our lives.

Maybe someday we'll actually have doctors who specialize in the care and treatment of the ocean inside us. Until then, we need to manage it ourselves.

# What Water Does

Our true watery nature can be hard to remember, but a 150-pound person is really twelve one-gallon milk jugs filled with water sitting next to a 50-pound bag of chemicals. That's a human being. When we're fetuses, we are about 75 percent water. That percentage is at its lowest when we're old—60 percent. So we can see how the trend goes. Wetter is better.

The water in our bodies exists in many forms. Around three-quarters of it is held inside the walls of our 70-plus trillion cells. And there are many different fluids flowing inside our bodies—about one and a third gallons of blood, plus the interstitial fluids around our cells, gastric juices, mucus, bile, saliva, lymph, and the fluid in our eyeballs and surrounding our brains and spinal cords, plus semen (some of us). All, essentially, water. It adds up.

The old view of water was that it was just filler, like packing material—the stuff that held all the solid materials and kept them from bumping into each other. Now we understand that water has a purpose, just like those solids do. Many purposes. It is not a nutrient, but it performs important functions in every system.

Still, we insist on thinking of ourselves as solid beings, although the dry ingredients are in the minority. It's just like our view of the planet we inhabit—Earth is about as much water as we are, but we think of it as rock-solid. It's not. We're not. We're fluid. But it's just too freaky to imagine ourselves that way. We look in the mirror and don't see liquid. We touch ourselves and feel solid. Water is a magician.

It's a simple, lightweight molecule, just two atoms of hydrogen and one of oxygen, and yet it can take on so many forms, exhibit so many strange properties unlike anything else on the planet. How can it be a liquid and yet create a surface and a shape that maintains the integrity of a drop? How does it defy gravity and travel up trees and plants, from the ground to the sky? How can a solid float on it, or a lizard walk on it? Even science can't fully explain.

Water is a big part of what makes us miraculous. It's a miracle hiding in plain sight, a miracle that's not just in your face—it *is* your face. And your skin. And your hair, your organs, your muscles (70 percent water), your fat, your bones (22 percent) and your marrow, your toenails and your brain and nervous system. A miracle that's all around us. It *is* us.

Water is involved in every system and every event in our bodies—nothing happens without it.

It's transportation. Everything in our bodies that moves from one place to another does so on water. Inside, we are a vast network of waterways with many tributaries and channels and streams. Water is the vehicle for every nutrient, hormone, chemical messenger, enzyme, electrolyte, and brain pulse.

It escorts food from our lips to our digestive tracts, breaking it down as it descends. Then, thanks to a process called hydrolysis, the electrical energy of water undoes the chemical bonds of nutrients contained in our food, making them available for our bodies to use. From our gut, blood (plasma is 92 percent water) carries those nutrients to our cells.

But the cells aren't just gaping open to take nutrition in. Thanks to yet another process, osmosis, the water in our cells and the water that surrounds them cooperate to get the nutrients past the membranes and inside—where all of life is carried out. Those cells are miniature oceans of salt water, containing all the chemicals that sustain us.

Inside our cells is where mineral salts, electrolytes, and water combine to create the electrical energy that fires up the mitochondria, the power plants of the cell. Everything we do—the spark of life itself—starts there. But not without water.

Water is the temperature control center of the body. It stores heat like a passive solar energy system. When necessary, water cools our bodies with perspiration or heats them through electrical energy.

Water is responsible for removing the waste matter produced in our cells. The processes that take place inside those walls—energy creation, metabolism—all leave behind debris of one kind or another. Water carries the detritus of life past the cell membrane, into our bloodstream, and on to our liver and kidneys, where it can be filtered. And then water carries the wastes right out of our bodies.

Water, in the form of synovial fluids, is the viscous cushion that keeps our joints from grinding and our spinal discs from rubbing. Gout is acute inflammatory arthritis of the joints. In a 2009 study performed by the Boston University School of Medicine, sufferers who drank five to eight glasses of water the day before an attack of gout had 40 percent less chance of its recurrence compared to those who drank only one glass.

Water operates our immune system. The white blood cells created in the bone marrow have to reach our tissues to fight off disease. Lymphatic fluid, which is about the same percentage water as blood plasma, carries toxic substances and carcinogens to the lymph nodes, where they can be destroyed. Even modest dehydration lowers the level of germ-fighting proteins in the saliva, according to a study by the Extremes Research Group, Bangor University, in the United Kingdom.

Our brains and nervous systems are nearly all water—85 and 98 percent, respectively. All the electrical events that happen in there, all those thoughts and messages that keep us alive in every way imaginable, the incredible complexity of the central nervous system—nearly all water. Look at your laptop. Now imagine a computer infinitely more complex, made almost completely of water. Unreal!

Think about the electricity that powers our bodies. It's what makes our hearts beat and our brains communicate. But there's no wiring. Instead, water carries the current inside the nerve canals. Those cells are essentially little batteries. What happens when your car battery loses its water? Dead. No more power. We're no different.

Water is important to our deepest, most mysterious selves, but also to all our surfaces—our skin, hair, eyes, nails. We are at our most beautiful when we are properly hydrated. (Ask any supermodel.) We even smell and taste better. These might sound like superficial reasons for drinking water, but when you're as beautiful as you can be, it's a sign that you're in great shape on the inside, too. In a 2007 study carried out at the University of Missouri–Columbia nursing school, even undetectable levels of underhydration can lower tissue oxygen, impair healing, and increase wound infection.

As much as we need water, we are constantly losing it. Through the vapor in every exhalation, which rids our bodies of waste gases. Through each drop of sweat, which cools us to the temperature where everything can function properly. Through the constant flow of tears and saliva, which keep our eyes and mouths and throats working. And of course, through the normal processes of elimination. Adults typically produce about a quart and a half of urine daily, with the bulk of production occurring in the daytime. We lose nearly another quart and a half more through our skin, depending on how much we sweat, and in our feces and our exhalations.

And, unlike fat, we don't store water in our bodies. It constantly flows through us, in and out, in a way that's almost tidal. We lose about three quarts of it a day. It makes sense that if water is so vital, our bodies would make replenishing the supply a continual priority, right?

Well, no. Our thirst mechanisms don't work that way. As a result, most of us aren't drinking nearly enough water.

That's putting it mildly. According to a survey conducted by the federal Centers for Disease Control, 7 percent of adults report no daily consumption of water. That's zero. Thirty-six percent of respondents said they drink a measly one to three cups a day, 35 percent drink four to seven cups, and 22 percent have the recommended eight cups or more, meaning four-fifths of us don't get sufficient water. And people over fifty-five, who really need it, get less water than those who are younger. The epidemiologist at the CDC who performed the study was so stunned that she thought she'd made a mistake, and went back to recheck the figures. Unfortunately, she was right.

To some, drinking too little water won't sound like the end of the world. Even scientists and doctors don't all agree that it's a reason for worry. But if water is so crucial to so many of our processes, how could a lack of it not be a bad thing?

# The Meaning of Cellular Dehydration

The lack of sufficient water actually has two possible causes.

One, as we've seen, is that we just don't consume enough of it. And it's not only that we fail to drink as much as we use up. Unhealthy eating adds to the problem. Consuming fresh, raw fruits and vegetables is a powerful influence on overall hydration, just as eating processed foods depletes our water supply. According to a study conducted by researchers from the University of Aberdeen, Scotland, plant-based food, because of the minerals and other nutrients it contains, hydrates us even more effectively than plain water or sports drinks.

The other reason for our underhydration is a little trickier: we drink water that isn't doing its job properly. It's water, but not the right kind. It's inside our bodies, but it doesn't enter our cell walls, where it is needed. We may have taken in so much water that we feel absolutely no sensation of thirst, and still we are dry—inside our cells, where it counts most. There are symptoms of that, but unfortunately we don't associate these symptoms with thirst. That's a real problem.

When we talk about not having enough water, we use the term

*dehydration*, but what we really mean is cellular dehydration, which is different from the way the word is commonly used. When we hear "dehydration," we think of the cartoon guy crawling across Death Valley under a broiling sun, with buzzards circling overhead. To us, dehydration is a life-threatening medical condition requiring immediate emergency treatment.

Cellular dehydration is something else. Unfortunately, it's a chronic, everyday condition for a lot of us. We haven't even been taught the meaning of it, or how to recognize the signs of it, let alone the potential for health problems.

As we've already said, all our cells, depending on the kind of tissue they constitute, are meant to contain a certain percentage of water. Cellular dehydration just means they contain less than they need to operate properly.

Monitoring all the various bodily water levels is the brain. And because the brain requires more water than any other organ, it's in its own self-interest to pay constant attention.

When the brain notices that the body's water level is getting low, here's what it does: it begins hoarding. Cells throughout the body will actually give up some of their water. The brain is a notorious worrier. And it's also a very selfish master. In all matters, the brain gets served first.

And so, for a while at least, the brain is satisfied. But then, even that organ's water level gets low. At this point, the signal that the body needs water is transmitted, meaning our mouths become dry.

We take this as the first symptom of thirst. But it's not—it's the last. A dry mouth doesn't mean we should drink something right away. It means we should have been drinking more all along. It means our cells have been underhydrated for a while. Each of our cells becomes unable to function properly when the water level becomes too low. The ratio of solid materials to fluid inside the cell begins to shift away from what it should be. Seventy trillion cells are now too dry. Inside these cells—not inside your mouth—is where the serious effects of dehydration are felt. The body robs

Peter to pay Paul in thousands upon thousands of trades, all to keep the top organ, the brain, hydrated while sacrificing the other organs, skin, health, energy levels, digestive health, immune health, and so on.

This is why the quality of the water we drink is so important. Because unfiltered water may contain particles that stress our cells. That's why drinking a lot of water isn't enough—it has to be the right kind.

Depending on the source of our water, it may contain chemicals, organic materials, heavy metals, PCBs, fluoride, chloride, and any number of other substances. This is important because our water isn't static—it's constantly moving in and out of our cells, transporting nutrients, messages, debris, and other stuff back and forth. But for the water to maintain that motion, the molecules of whatever solids and/or electrolytes are suspended in it must be small. Otherwise, they can't pass through the openings in our cell membranes. The presence of particles is expressed as water's total dissolved solids (TDS) score. High TDS means there is potential to create debris that the cell must then handle. Usually, you want water that is 0–15ppm TDS. Distilled water is about 0–5.

That's why the form our nutrients take is as important as their nutritional value itself. If the molecules of the minerals, for instance, are too large, they'll never fit into our cells. Rather than nourish us, they'll just clog up the works and cause more cellular stress. It's just one more reason for eating whole, unprocessed foods, which are dependably bioavailable. Our bodies can get at them.

The same is true for the electrolytes and other supposedly healthy ingredients contained in sports and vitamin drinks. Electrolytes are minerals that conduct electricity in a solution— the main ones are sodium, potassium, calcium, and magnesium. We need them in order to live. But the molecules have to be small enough to do our cells any good. Any bigger than an angstrom, and it's like trying to shove a basketball into a garden hose.

Makers of sports drinks like to spout scientific-sounding boasts about their products, but we must consider the source. A team of scientists at Oxford University examined 431 claims made in 104 advertisements and concluded that there's a "worrying" lack of high-quality studies on the effects of sports drinks and protein shakes. It's even possible to overdo them, something the manufacturers won't tell you. In 2003 the Texas Medical Association Council on Scientific Affairs published a report stating that the "abuse of sports drinks may result in adverse effects." It cited the case of a football player who took in a whopping 5 grams of potassium a day from a drink meant to restore salts lost in perspiration. As a result he suffered potassium-induced cardiac arrhythmia.

This is why any drink but clean, or vortated, filtered spring water should be avoided. Other beverages may quench our thirst, but we don't know if they can hydrate us at the cellular level, where it counts. If we fill up on low-quality beverages, we won't be thirsty enough to drink good water, should it come along.

Even stress contributes to cellular dehydration. All forms of stress—emotional, nutritional—stimulate the production of cortisol, known as the stress hormone. This shuts down normal metabolism and draws water from our cells in a process called diffusion. Diuretic, processed foods, including caffeinated drinks like coffee, tea, and some sodas, do the same, as does excessive protein consumption. This becomes yet another harmful cycle—stress causes dehydration, which leads to more stress. Two studies conducted by the University of Connecticut's Human Performance Laboratory found even mild dehydration caused worsening of mood and made tasks seem more difficult.

# How to Tell You Need Water

What exactly happens when our cells are underhydrated? Nothing we notice as such.

When our cells first become underhydrated, we may feel tired. But who associates fatigue with dehydration? They are linked, though. When your cells don't have enough water, your body's response is to slow everything down by slowing the endocrine system. According to a 2010 review of previous research, which appeared in the British Nutrition Foundation's *Nutrition Bulletin*, "Dehydration resulting in loss of body mass of 2 percent or more can result in reduced physical performance, headaches and symptoms of fatigue."

Thus we feel weary when it's not bedtime. Pretty common. Our typical response? Maybe a cup of coffee or a soda with caffeine. Maybe something to eat that's full of sugar and simple carbs, like a granola bar or a doughnut. This does nothing for our hydration. If anything, it makes things worse as our bodies try to cope with the hit of caffeine and sugar, both of which use up water in order to process. And we're getting addicted to the sugary taste (even if it was sugar-free soda), or the chemical hit of caffeine, or the sedation of alcohol, making us even less inclined to want water next time we're thirsty.

We each create our own internal water environment, and our bodies adapt to it. If we drink two ounces of water a day, our bodies will figure a way to exist on that. We won't die. But we won't be healthy. The human body can adapt to almost any deprivation we throw at it. It's the secret to our survival as a species, but you could say that's also a disadvantage. We're so adaptable that we manage to survive on less water than is good for us.

We won't know it, but cell dehydration is creating many unfavorable internal conditions. Every fluid in our bodies becomes sludgy. We're not eliminating wastes as well as we should. Our immune systems are slower to respond than normal. We're less able to create mucous membrane, which means our digestive tracts will suffer. All enzymatic function will lessen, making our bodies more acidic, which then creates its own new set of problems.

None of this sounds very good in the short run, but imagine what happens when we are in a chronic state of underhydration.

I don't mean for just a day or two or a week or a month, either. I'm talking about years—decades—of not having sufficient water for our bodies to function optimally. Which is how it usually goes. As we've noted, the older we get, the less water we drink.

Here's what can result from chronic cellular dehydration.

Cancer and hypertension—two of the modern age's biggest killers.

Our kidneys' ability to regulate blood pressure can be harmed by insufficient hydration. What science refers to as "low drinkers"—people who take in less water than recommended—produce higher than normal levels of arginine vasopressin (AVP), a hormone that tells the kidneys to conserve body water. Low drinkers show evidence of this and other physiological adaptations to conserve total body water and maintain normal water content in blood plasma. Also, when we are underhydrated, our blood volume lessens due to the lack of water in the plasma. To compensate, our blood vessels constrict. Our heart rate increases, too. Elevated AVP may also cause an increased risk of hyperglycemia—excessive blood sugar.

In addition, the low urine volumes observed in low drinkers may have long-term implications for kidney health, potentially including an increased risk of chronic kidney disease. All the kidneys' various functions require us to drink the recommended amounts of water.

If we don't get enough water, our bodies can't eliminate cellular debris, which may damage our DNA. Dehydration has a negative impact on our telomeres, which leads to unhealthy aging and even an increased risk of cancer. Fluctuations in water level can also damage the mechanism that controls cell shape, a hallmark for development of metastatic cancers. A lack of water causes histamine production to increase, which shuts down the release of interferon, a critical anti-cancer chemical that is present in a hydrated body. Histamine suppresses immune activity in the bone marrow, which is where we produce the white blood cells that digest and destroy cancer cells.

Water deficit is the primary cause of many other disease symptoms too. Chronic pain, digestive distress, migraines, depression—all may be attributed at least partly to a lack of cellular hydration. The same is true for all the degenerative diseases. We are literally dying of thirst. But when we ask doctors for help, they don't even consider this possibility, because they haven't been taught the importance of water to health. Instead, they go directly to prescription painkillers or other drugs that not only may not address the problem but can actually worsen it, adding to the burden on our overburdened bodies.

"Dehydration of as little as 1 percent decrease in body weight results in impaired physiological and performance responses," according to a 1999 article in the *Journal of the American Dietetic Association*. For a 150-pound person, this is merely a pound and a half of water weight. "New research indicates that fluid consumption in general and water consumption in particular can have an effect on the risk of urinary stone disease; cancers of the breast, colon, and urinary tract; childhood and adolescent obesity; mitral valve prolapse; salivary gland function; and overall health in the elderly."

Dehydration leads to enzymatic and hormonal changes that damage or destroy our cellular receptors, those structures that allow cells to receive nutrition and information from other parts of the body. When cells can't accept communications, they become isolated from their environment, and the chance that they will become sick increases.

When our histamine level rises due to insufficient hydration, we begin to react to allergens in the air that we might otherwise ignore. Suddenly we have all the typical symptoms of allergies—even to natural substances in the air and food, in addition to industrial toxins and irritants. In reality, we're not allergic at all. Our bodies are simply responding to a lack of cellular water.

A 2002 study by the Division of Wellness and Chronic Illness, State University of New York—Stony Brook, discovered that patients with asthma and allergic rhinitis as well as other chronic allergies improved with proper hydration and balanced nutrition. In his 2003 book *Water: For Health, for Healing, for Life; You're Not Sick, You're Thirsty!*, Dr. Fereydoon Batmanghelidj observed that chronic dehydration prompts the body to prevent respiratory water loss by producing histamines, which close off lung capillaries and increase the likelihood of allergic reactions.

Headaches are also linked to cell dehydration. In surveys, more than one-third of migraine sufferers report that dehydration can provoke their attacks, "a precipitant not recognized by the medical profession," according to a 2005 article in the medical journal *Headache*.

Research has associated many psychological problems with insufficient water. We've all been taught that our emotional disorders are due to nonphysical causes best treated (and treated, and treated) by mental health professionals. But often they are triggered by a simple lack of hydration. When our brains are starved for water, they stop functioning properly—not surprisingly, considering that they are 85 percent $H_2O$.

Researchers at Tufts University found that student athletes who engaged in hard exercise and failed to drink enough water were more likely to report feeling depressed, tense, confused, angry, and tired than those who exercised but drank. The lesson here applies to us all, not just young athletes.

In a study conducted at the University of Connecticut's Human Performance Laboratory, mild dehydration was induced in a group of women. The lack of water led to fatigue, headaches, and dampened moods. They also reported that tasks seemed more difficult, and they had problems concentrating. Once they were properly hydrated, all the complaints disappeared.

I tell people this all the time: if you feel tired or cranky or down during the day, don't have coffee, tea, or soda—drink a big glass of water, and see how you feel. Most people are energized by it. Suddenly, their mood lifts.

ADHD, too, is affected by hydration. Our neurological receptors malfunction when our cells go thirsty. A recent study determined that two-thirds of children show up for school every day slightly dehydrated. They either don't drink anything when they wake up, or they drink juice or some other liquid that contains sodium or amino acids (like milk), leaving their cells even less hydrated. Once the children in the study had a single glass of water, they were retested, and their academic performance instantly improved. Imagine the long-term effect of cell dehydration on young brains and their intellectual ability.

Kids who were underhydrated also showed an impaired aptitude for remembering numbers. Don't you think the "epidemic" of ADHD might have something to do with a child's inability to focus on schoolwork, caused by something as simple as not enough water?

Bloating? Doctors will try and treat water retention with drugs. But it's a sign of dehydration—your body wants to retain what water it has left, so the cells secrete sodium, which just makes you even more dehydrated.

Arthritis, joint pain, skin problems—all are signs that your body is rationing water, sparing it for what's absolutely necessary, so your skin and your joints suffer. Bacteria and viruses that collect on our surfaces can easily penetrate dry, cracked skin. Our skin isn't just a cosmetic covering—it's the first line of defense in our immune systems. Insufficiently hydrated, it can't do that job.

We're constipated. And we can't figure out why. We have colitis, gastritis, arthritis, extreme PMS, diverticulitis, and other digestive problems. These all might stem from a lack of water at the cellular level—to the point where nothing in our bodies functions as it should. Clearly, the lack of water is causing havoc inside us. Dehydration is our bodies' number-one stressor. No other single factor has the potential to cause so many illnesses and do us so much harm.

We all constantly bitch about the cost of medical care and health insurance, and here we have a guaranteed illness-prevention method that is virtually free. We can avoid so many disorders and diseases, even serious ones, even fatal ones, just by drinking a few extra glasses of water a day. Can it be any simpler? Any cheaper?

But how could we not know all this? Medical science still treats us based on discoveries made a long time ago. We're living in the twenty-first century, and doctors see us through a nineteenth-century lens. There's something wrong with our joints, or our heart, or our skin, or our glands. And so there's a sub-subspecialty to treat us.

The problem's not necessarily with our individual parts, though; maybe it's with our water. All our ailments are the result of systemwide deficiencies. We know that now, but health care hasn't caught up. Because of that outdated approach, our bodies and minds are needlessly suffering. Look at all the signature diseases of modern life: high blood pressure, high cholesterol, arthritis, diabetes, allergies, osteoporosis. In every case, the "solution" is a pill we need to take every day for the rest of our lives.

Whenever doctors and scientists discuss the health of any body part or organ—our livers, our joints, our brains—they focus on the solid matter, the tissues, the structures, without paying attention to the water, even though water is a major part of whatever it is they're discussing. Water is ignored because it's too mysterious and impossible to pin down. It makes scientists uneasy, but it's always there.

What if instead of always treating our organs as though there's something wrong with them, we first consider the state of the water they contain, or even just ask if there's enough of it? Why not look at the largest single component of our bodies as the possible source of ill health, rather than always blaming this organ or that one? Or, what if it's the water surrounding our organs that has the greatest effect on them? Maybe your body is sick because it's a desert inside. Sometimes the simplest things can heal the gnarliest problems. Like drinking water. But we have to do it.

Even the people who devote themselves to the study of water end up admitting they barely understand it.

# Water and Me

As you may have noticed, I'm passionate about water. There's a reason that I grew up in Minnesota but ended up in Malibu, and it's not only the weather.

But when I was young, water was just water. Something you drink when you're thirsty. Even playing college football, we didn't think much about it. Once I learned that our brains and nervous systems and muscles were mostly water, I started carrying a big plastic jug of it around with me. It was spring water, according to the label, and that was good enough for me. I certainly wasn't worried about anything further, including the possibility that PCBs and other chemicals in those plastic bottles could be leaching into what I drank.

Then I read somewhere that drinking distilled water was a healthier way to go, so I made the switch. I used to train bodybuilders, and I was accustomed to using distilled water to pull the excess salt out of someone's body to help make competition weight. (Crazy, I know.)

A week of that, a gallon a day, definitely made me leaner. But I started feeling lousy. Because distilled water is pH-neutral, it had no electrolytes and was pulling needed salts out of my cells, just like it pulled them from those bodybuilders. Definitely not a good idea, because over time it takes a toll. At the time I was still eating meat, and I needed all the alkalinity I could get. So I went back to spring water, felt better immediately, and didn't give it another thought.

I went along that way until I began talking to people who were studying water in a serious way and coming up with some surprising results. Like how the pipes that water passes through can affect its molecular shape and its frequency. Or how chemicals from its container can adulterate it and change it. Today these ideas are generally accepted, but that wasn't always the case.

The Japanese take water seriously. They've been studying it for centuries. There, Masaru Emoto tried an interesting experiment. He labeled containers of water with different words, froze them, and then photographed the resulting ice crystals using a special camera. The crystal structure actually changed, he claimed, depending on the meaning of the words. His discovery got lots of attention, of course, not all of it favorable. Many doubt the significance of what he found, but no one has been able to explain it away.

The fact is that water is changed, and can be manipulated, by everything that touches it. There are a number of terms for this—structured water, functional water. They all mean essentially the same thing: that water is sensitive to outside influences, beneficial or otherwise.

Researchers have treated water with light to see how its molecule structure changes, or charged it electrically to alter its pH, which increases its health benefits, making it better at fighting cancer and degenerative diseases. These researchers' claims have been disputed, but that's just more proof of the continuing mystery of water and its ability to shape-shift. Merely by agitating it with a silver or copper spoon before we drink it, we may alter its properties for the better. The color of its container changes water, too. Colors have frequencies; it makes sense that water would be influenced by the frequency surrounding it.

I tend to be open to all kinds of possibilities where water's concerned, in case you haven't guessed. I believe water absorbs messages—positive, negative, life affirming, soul destroying, whatever we send, whatever touches us. All that water inside us, listening, being enhanced or degraded by our own thoughts and feelings and experiences. What happens to us happens to our water. Our water's fate is our fate, too.

It's no different from the relationship between the health of the seas and that of the planet. Changes in the oceans change everything on land—the temperature, the weather, the air quality, the food. We know that our planet depends on the health of its oceans, and that the oceans depend on humans not defiling them with so much pollution that they become sick. Sick oceans, sick planet. And in just the same way, if our water is sick, so are we.

I don't need the AMA to tell me how important water is to my well-being. I don't require a ton of scientific journals to affirm and reaffirm a fact before I am ready to test-drive it.

I'm in awe of water. I really do think it is one of the most mysteriously powerful forces on the planet. Does that sound crazy? Through all the millennia that we've been on this planet, one thing after another has sounded crazy at first. And some of them turned out to be absolute truth. Maybe someday we'll learn enough about water to explain how it can be like a blank canvas, or a computer's hard drive, retaining a memory of everything it touches.

When astrophysicists wonder if other planets can support life, they always ask first: Is there water? Water equals life. Water does exist elsewhere in the universe, in frozen form; life, however, seems to depend on it being liquid. How can one simple molecule be responsible for so much that goes on in our bodies, in all living things, and even in our world?

We don't have to completely understand water. We just have to acknowledge its power. How do we do this?

By drinking a lot of it. How much? People use all kinds of formulas. One ounce of water for every two pounds of body weight is a good rule. If we don't feel like doing the arithmetic, somewhere between three and four liters a day is probably enough. Here's another good rule of thumb: After your first pee of the day, your urine should be either clear or pale yellow. If it's darker than that, you probably aren't getting enough water.

The important thing is that we drink more than our thirst response seems to require. We need to make sure that we never feel thirsty. The more we drink, the more our bodies will use, and so the more we will crave it, which is a very good thing. If you drink from a glass, you should always have one filled. If you use a bottle, it should always be at hand.

And it needs to be water itself. Obviously, any drink is mostly water, but we're not getting the benefit of it when we consume other beverages. Even the commercially available bottled waters that supposedly contain vitamins and other things aren't as good as clean water, with only natural minerals.

We use up water as we sleep. First thing in the morning, our tank is low; we need a refill. In fact, the first meal of the day should be water—a liter is a healthy way to start the morning, and if we throw in a pinch of unrefined crystal salt, a pinch of cayenne pepper, and a squirt of fresh lemon juice, we have a great jump-start that prepares our digestion, hydrates us, and opens up proper secretions for detoxing.

Remember that study of schoolchildren and water—it makes us smarter. We should all be smarter.

Our mastery of water is so total that we hardly notice it. Wherever we go, there are taps. Twist one, and out comes clean water, hot or cold as we choose, so abundant it's virtually infinite. Things are different in other parts of the world. When I tell people there that we flush our toilets with clean water, they shake their heads in awe; they can't imagine such a thing. Plenty of people still die due to a lack of clean water. There are 400 million kids on this planet without free access to clean water.

We take water for granted, and then we render that water unsafe to drink. We allow dangerous levels of chemical pollutants, toxic chemicals, organic substances, and dissolved solids in our tap water. We kill off most of the illness-causing microbes, but we do it with chemicals like chloride and fluoride, which shouldn't be ingested. Other technologies exist that could do the same job safely, but they're not widely accepted yet. We could even have systems in our own homes to make drinking water safe, giving us some control over the chemicals we consume every day.

We manage to take some of the bad chemicals out of our water, but then our heavy pharmaceutical habit repollutes it. We toss out billions of prescription pills and capsules, which eventually end up in our taps. Cities routinely test for this, finding every drug imaginable—even the illegal ones. It's gotten so bad that there are government campaigns to get people to stop flushing their unused medicines down the toilet. But we still do it. Even the drugs we swallow end up in the water supply, when our bodies eliminate their residue.

The chemicals used every day in industry also find their way into our water. Do we know the long-term effects of every new chemical? Of course we don't. We take them in blindly and cross our fingers.

In 2009 the Environmental Working Group did analyses of drinking water throughout the United States, and discovered hundreds of pollutants in tap water. The most common chemicals were arsenic, nitrate, fertilizers, and trihalomethanes, which can cause cancer. A study conducted at the School of Public Health of Taipei Medical University in 2000 found that long-term consumption of chlorine and trihalomethanes in tap water can increase the risk of cancer.

Our drinking water contains what the government considers "acceptable" levels of dissolved solids, chemicals, pesticides, medications, radiation, putrefaction, human and animal wastes, and other organic materials. Water picks up a little of everything it touches. That's why science calls it "the universal solvent." It has a memory of everything it has ever experienced, even energy.

Meaning there's no such thing as "pure" water. It's all tea.

This is why I advise people: Do not drink tap water. I don't care where it's from, or how good it's supposed to be. It's so important to drink water that has touched only the right things. When it comes from unpolluted springs, it has been exposed to oxygen due to its movement through the earth. As it rushes over rocks and dirt, it picks up minerals and salts. The sunlight infuses it with healthy energy. Movement, minerals, and the sun all structure water naturally, making it more biologically harmonious to our cells and body.

But I don't live near an unspoiled mountain spring. Maybe you do. If not, then we both have to figure a way to get the water we need from the world we inhabit.

You can try bottled spring water. But of course we still have no way of knowing what exactly that water contains. We don't know what happened to it on the way from the spring. We do know that being held for weeks or months in a plastic bottle isn't making it any healthier. That's why I think we should steer clear of commercially produced bottled spring water, too.

Where does that leave us? Distilled water. That, in my view, is the safe way to go—the only truly clean water. Low TDS of 0–5 ppm; pH neutral, 7.0. Not the most convenient solution, I agree. But with something as vital as water, convenience may have to take a back seat to health.

We can buy distilled water in huge jugs—you can get it delivered to your home—and then immediately pour it into a glass container or water cooler. Or we can try tabletop water distillers, which are easily found online, machines that heat water and then collect the vapor and eliminate everything else.

My own solution may be a bit more elaborate than you're ready to try. I own a machine that pulls vapor from the air, condenses it into liquid, and then filters it extremely well. The device costs thousands of dollars. To me, it's well worth it. My whole life is devoted to finding the very best, cleanest, highest-quality foods on the planet, so I couldn't cut corners when it comes to water.

Distilled water has been stripped of its impurities along with everything else, even good things, like minerals, so we need to add them back in. Half a teaspoon of unprocessed crystal salt to a gallon of water does the trick. Or a pinch of salt in a twelve-ounce glass. If possible, use unrefined Himalayan crystal salt; formed 250 million years ago beneath the surface of the earth, it is as clean as salt can be. Because it's unprocessed, it still contains all the minerals and trace elements that support good health. The molecules are also the right size to enter our cells.

That salt will make the water slightly alkaline, which is what we want. Do not drink distilled or condensed water without adding salt, or your body will give up minerals to balance the water, which can lead to deficiencies.

Finally, when you drink that water, think kindly of it. Be grateful for it. And—because when you drink, you are instantly replenishing your own flesh and blood—above all, love your water.

I keep my water in a cobalt-blue glass bottle that sunlight can pass through. Water is a conductor of energy, storing some of the sun's radiant power and passing it along to me. I have the word GRATITUDE etched into the glass, because I am grateful for my water, and I believe that expressing that gratitude matters. Water absorbs emotion as it absorbs everything else that touches it. I realize how nutty that may sound, but I don't mind. Is there any scientific proof that a word written on a bottle will make me healthier? Define *proof*. There is enough evidence for me to know that the water that goes inside me is as important as the water that's already there. I respect water because it contains answers to mysteries about our bodies that science still hasn't touched.

# Simple To-Do List

✓

- We spend eight hours or so daily without drinking a single drop—when we sleep. We need to start every morning with a big glass of water to replace what we've lost during the night.

- Our kids also need to drink lots of water, especially before school in the morning. The latest research has found that their test scores and academic abilities actually depend on whether or not they've been drinking enough water.

- Drink pure water only. Commercially bottled water with vitamins or other added substances often contain sugars, which degrade our health at worst. At best, the additives are not beneficial.

- Make the extra effort to drink only filtered, distilled water to which we have added the unrefined salts our bodies require. It's work but it's worth it.

- Drink a big glass of water when you feel tired, fuzzy-brained or emotionally drained. I'm betting that most of the time, water will be just what you needed.

# The Big Fix Syndrome

If an alien came from another planet and observed how we manage our nutritional lives, he would come to one obvious conclusion: a lot of humans have no interest in being healthy. He'd figure that we are cool with heart disease, cancer, diabetes, arthritis; that we don't mind indigestion, obesity, stinky breath, dry skin, achy joints, flabby bellies; that we're on some kind of self-destructive trip—practically suicidal. What other conclusion could that alien possibly reach? Given our actions, we must *want* to be sick.

Maybe that's because once we actually *get* sick, we're on familiar ground. Now we know what to do. We call in the heavyweight help: Big Medicine.

An interesting thing about pharmaceuticals is that about 90 percent of them are based on or inspired by substances contained in plants. What does that tell us? That even the laboratory must turn to nature to learn how to heal us.

Another interesting thing about prescription pharmaceuticals is that, by latest count, around 70 percent of Americans are taking at least one. Seven out of ten of us take an expensive synthesized version of something that probably exists in food. But it's easier to swallow a pill. We make up 5 percent of the world's population, and we take 80 percent of all prescription painkillers. Are we in so much more pain than everybody else, or is it that the rest of the world is content to live in chronic misery? Or is there a third possibility: that we're just in love with drugs? After all, they are the solution we trust and have come to expect.

Are we at least getting good results? According to the latest World Health Organization figures available, the United States is ranked thirty-fourth in the world for life expectancy. There are a lot of ties on the list, so in truth there are more than thirty-three other countries where the average citizen lives longer than we Americans do. Actually, I should say we U.S. citizens, since Chile, Canada, and Costa Rica have a higher life expectancy, as do Japan (number one) and most western European and Scandinavian countries. We come in right below Bahrain and above Cuba.

Just above *Cuba*? Does that make you wonder?

Medications, even when they help us, take a toll on the body. They're a challenge to digest and metabolize. They acidify our tissues. They stress and tax all our systems. Medicine may some-times be a miracle, but it always has its costs. There is a waterfall of side effects, which require other pharmaceuticals to neutralize them. It's like a merry-go-round—once you get on, it's hard to get off.

The biggest failure, however, especially of drugs for chronic conditions such as heart disease, high blood pressure, arthritis, diabetes, and so on, is this: these medicines don't cure anything.

If they cured us, we could stop taking them. But they don't, and so we can't. They muffle the symptoms. They mask the problem. They treat the disease, but not the person, and certainly not the nutritional deficiency.

We don't merely take these drugs until the illness goes away, because the illness never goes away.

The drugs just allow us to live without going to all the trouble of changing our habits and fixing what's really wrong. They allow us to be somewhat functional and yet chronically unwell. Pseudo-functional. They make it possible for us to go on like that until the day—way down the road, of course—when our unhealthy habits fi-nally catch up with us and even medicine can't help.

When that happens, well . . . let's not even think about it.

Here is the terrible deal that our civilization cuts us: We may eat poorly and not exercise, but we can still live and be somewhat okay—as long as we take our medicine.

This, I guess, is the medical-industrial complex at work.

With our eager cooperation, food manufacturers and restaurant chains and fast-food giants get rich by making us sick. Then the pharmaceutical giants and the insurance companies and hospitals and other health care providers get rich by making us better. Not healthy, mind you, but well enough to work and pay the bills we've just run up.

If we ate our broccoli and quinoa and salads and berries and almonds and drank our water and green tea and took long, vigorous hikes and got enough sleep, we might feel great, but who would profit? Nobody. What kind of system is that?

When something is wrong with us, drugs should be the last resort, not the first. Rather than sending us to the pharmacy with prescriptions, our physicians should send us to the farmers' market with shopping lists. Instead of spending billions to develop and promote the next wonder drug, the pharmaceutical giants could just grow the plants that yield the food containing those substances in their natural form.

But it's more glamorous to be a scientist than a farmer, I guess. Pays better, too. It's easier to work at a desk in a nice, clean, air-conditioned lab than it is to drive a tractor in a hot dirt field. There's a bigger profit margin in Crestor than cranberries.

We keep hearing how the problem with preventive medicine is that it doesn't work as a business model for health care. But that's only because we're willing to pay more to treat an illness with drugs than to avoid it with food. Maybe making a change would require a total transformation of the system, but that sounds like a good thing to me. Systems need transforming when they don't do their job.

In poor countries, of course, it's different. Most people can't afford the drugs and the hospitals and the surgery. They can't even afford the abundant food and clean drinking water we enjoy. So they need to be very, very careful when it comes to their health. How do they manage this?

First, they recognize that food is a kind of medicine. Actually, that's an insult—to food. Food is much better than medicine. It's cheaper, safer, more easily absorbed, and tastes better. Even socially, food is superior. I never heard of a family or friends sitting around a table together taking their medicine.

People in the undeveloped world understand that food has healing powers. It doesn't exist just to fill their bellies—it is their anti-inflammatory, their antioxidant, their multivitamin. And so they make sure to eat and drink the right things.

In India, most people cook with the spice turmeric every day. It's what makes curry yellow. It is a staple of Indian cuisine and has been for centuries. Curcumin, a phytonutrient present in turmeric, is a potent anti-inflammatory, good for the immune, glandular, and endocrine systems, as well as joint health—quite a godsend. Add a little pepper, and curcumin becomes even more effective. If you go into any store that sells nutritional supplements, you will find curcumin in pill form. Without knowing anything about the particular brand your store sells, I can practically guarantee that the curcumin found in turmeric is of better quality—purer, more natural, and more bio-available.

I've visited turmeric fields in India and met farmers whose families have grown it for six and seven generations. It would never occur to them to disrespect their crop by turning it into something other than a delicious spice that has kept them healthy for centuries. They are connected to their food and its healing possibilities in a way that we seem to have lost. They don't wait until they are sick to start eating turmeric—they consume it every day, starting in childhood, knowing that it will help protect them from infection and disease. They don't have to read a study published in the *Journal of the American Medical Association* to convince them to eat it.

If you can't afford or don't have ready access to drugs to treat illness, it becomes extremely important to eat in a way that prevents it. For some reason, our ability to pay for antibiotics and anti-inflammatories and all the rest has made disease prevention much less of a priority. It's weird. Who wants to be sick if it's avoidable? We do, I guess, judging by our behaviors. It would sure seem that way to a Martian.

# The Exercise Factor:

*Here's Your Ferrari*

Strictly speaking, physical movement—exercise, activity, whatever you want to call it—isn't a nutrient.

But it's as important as any of them. It literally activates our bodies. We eat and drink to fuel life—not just existence but active living and doing all that our bodies can do. Otherwise, what's the point? It would be like having that Ferrari and never driving it.

We don't have to be scientists to figure out what a human body is built to do. Any six-year-old could come up with the list. We've evolved into beings who are really excellent at walking, running, jumping, climbing, pushing, pulling, bending, stretching, lifting, and carrying. We are capable of exerting great explosive power. We are quick and agile. Even compared to wild animals, we have incredible endurance.

All this seems obvious, and once you study us in detail—how our brains and nervous systems operate, how our skeletons and muscles function, the complex way our bodies use nutrition to fuel our actions—it only becomes clearer: We are amazing creatures who are made to move.

For most of our time on this planet, that's what we did. When we were hunters and gatherers, we walked. A lot. We ran for our lives at times, defended our families, maybe chased down dinner now and then. When we found what we were looking for, we picked it up and carried it home. Then, just ten thousand or so years ago, we became farmers, but we still walked and lifted and built things and worked hard. It wasn't by choice. We depended on our physical strength to survive.

But our brains were powerful, too. It seems like human nature to want to make life easier, to spare ourselves the stress and danger of physical labor. This wish makes perfect sense. Who wants a life of crushing hard work? Civilization has pretty much devoted itself to this single goal: to ease the burden of survival and give us time and energy for other things. Fun things, even.

This is wonderful, right?

Of course, there's no stopping civilization once it gets going. Who could have anticipated that what would benefit us would also harm us?

We have taken nearly all the mandatory physical exertion out of our daily lives. Hurray for us—it really is a great achievement.

Unfortunately, we're suffering because of it, too.

Current studies say that most people get no regular exercise.

None.

Zero.

That's crazy! We invented exercise because we were no longer moving or exerting our bodies. We all know we should do it, just like we know we should eat our vegetables and fruit, drink lots of water, and get plenty of sleep. But that doesn't seem to be enough to get us moving.

Today, endless scientific studies prove what we already know: physical activity is good for us. But still, it's persuasive when you see in detail how it changes us. For example . . .

According to several studies, people who engage in regular exercise live three to seven years longer than those who don't. It lowers the production of C-reactive protein, which means decreased inflammation, which in turn means lower risk of heart attack and cancer. The physical duress of exercise stimulates the short-term release of the so-called stress hormone, cortisol, which is normal. But activity then lowers the long-term production of this hormone—which is a good thing, since chronically high levels of cortisol have been linked to a long list of disorders, including a weakened immune system, high blood pressure, lower bone density, depression, and increased blood sugar.

Exercise makes our tissues more sensitive to insulin, meaning we are less likely to develop type 2 diabetes. We probably won't become overweight due to metabolic syndrome either. And even if we do, exercise may come to the rescue. A study from the Norwegian University of Science and Technology reported that subjects with metabolic syndrome who followed a sixteen-week program of high-intensity interval training had a 100 percent greater decrease in the fat-producing enzyme fatty acid synthase than subjects who followed continuous moderate-intensity workouts.

Exercise lowers estrogen and progesterone in the bloodstream; elevated levels of both those hormones have been linked to uterine cancer. A study by the School of Sport, Exercise and Health Sciences at Loughborough University in Leicestershire, England, suggests that vigorous exercise suppresses the key hunger hormone ghrelin for up to thirty minutes after workouts, and increases levels of the appetite-suppressing hormone peptide YY for as long as three hours after exercise. That's a twofer.

A study at the University of Texas Southwestern Medical Center tested mice's rate of autophagy—a process that recycles cellular debris by burning it for energy—based on whether or not the mice exercised. The rate increased in the creatures who were forced to work out. This is especially important because autophagy is partly responsible for how well or badly we age. The implication is clear: physical activity keeps us young.

Our bodies adapt to the stress of exercise by making us healthier—our muscles and bones become stronger, our hearts and arteries more capable, our lungs more efficient in delivering oxygen to our tissues. But the increased consumption of oxygen actually has one downside—it causes oxidative stress, meaning damage done by free radicals. This is easily countered, however, by eating a diet containing plenty of antioxidant fruits and vegetables. It all works together, every system, every life force.

A study by researchers from the Dana-Farber Cancer Institute and Harvard Medical School shows how physical activity improves us at the cellular level. Exercise, they found, stimulates production of a previously unknown hormone that may turn our unhealthy white fat into beneficial brown fat, making us less likely to become obese or develop diabetes and other metabolic sicknesses.

A 2013 paper published in the scientific journal *PLOS Genetics* shows how exercise changes us even at our most fundamental level: our DNA. Researchers at the Lund University Diabetes Centre in Sweden discovered that exercise affects the cells that cluster around our genes, altering how they express proteins. As a result, the risk for obesity or type 2 diabetes is lowered. And the scientists found that these changes begin to take place after just one workout.

We could go on this way all day, study upon study, but the point would be the same: exercise improves us at all levels, from the cosmetic to the cellular. It makes us stronger in every sense of the word.

The weird part is that while science keeps proving how exercise will help us live longer and healthier, we respond by getting less of it. Common sense says that we will take actions that benefit us and avoid ones that hurt us. In most aspects of our lives, that's how we operate. But not when it comes to the most important part of life—our health. It's hard to figure.

My motivation was simple: I picked up my first dumbbell at age sixteen because I was scrawny and tired of being picked on by my older brother. And it did the trick. I became strong enough to play football in college. I haven't stopped working out since. If we keep making choices that challenge us, we will always be rewarded.

Even evolution has provided us with a great motivation to exercise. We've all heard of the "runner's high"—the physical pleasure caused when exertion prompts the release of endorphins in our brains. These neurotransmitters are like a natural narcotic, like heroin that's good for us.

But evolution also seems to offer an explanation for why we shun challenging activity. Back when we were still in caves and lived a subsistence lifestyle, we worked when we had to, and otherwise we rested. We needed that rest! Life consisted of short periods of hard physical labor and long stretches of lying around relaxing, the anthropologists tell us.

Look at wild animals today, and you'll see how we might have been then. Lions hang around doing nothing for as long as possible, and then they spring into action when they're hungry. It's the hunger that motivates the action. They don't chase zebras because they think they need more cardio.

We're no different. Our bodies don't want us to burn any more energy than is necessary. Why do you think we store it in the form of fat? That's how we managed to survive as a species when nutrition was scarce. Back then, voluntary exercise would have been self-destructive. Even just a few generations ago, most people did hard physical labor all day. They didn't need treadmills or gym memberships to make sure they got their workout.

Now food is in constant abundance. We can eat all we want with virtually no energy output required to gather it—just a quick drive to the supermarket or the doughnut shop. Without the motivation of hunger, activity has become an entirely voluntary thing.

And there are way too few volunteers.

Is there any hope for changing this? Trying to guilt people into exercising doesn't work. President Kennedy encouraged us to get more activity sixty years ago. Since then, we've gotten less. Making people feel bad about not exercising may end up discouraging them from even trying.

I think there's an unnoticed cause-and-effect between our worsening diet and our increasing inactivity. Exercise requires fuel. When we eat improperly, will our bodies feel much like moving around? When we're acidic, underhydrated, and lacking in the nutrients that our brains, bones, and muscles need, will we crave physical challenges or just a nice soft couch and a big-screen TV?

If we lack the desire to move and challenge our muscles, one reason has to be because we're not getting all the nutrients and water needed to keep us healthy. The mere fact that we don't want to be active is a symptom of some underlying deficiency. It's a sign that something is wrong. A healthy body is active.

Now, reconsider the statistic that the majority of people don't get any regular exercise. The reason suddenly comes into focus: we're eating worse than ever, and we're moving less than ever, and those two scary facts are tightly linked. Most people today don't have the strength or the energy for hard physical effort.

No animal was created to sit around and do nothing. There's no such thing as stillness, not even in our bodies. Inside, we are in perpetual motion. The flow of information inside our bodies, from cell to cell, is constant. In nature, stagnation equals dysfunction and disease and death.

On the other hand, if we feed our cells what they need, and we give our bones and muscles the power to burst into action, and our hearts and lungs are capable of responding to great physical challenges, will we be content lying around doing nothing?

No way. Once we get the keys to that Ferrari and gas it up, we'll be ready to *go*.

# Exercise and the Five Life Forces

I've been working out hard since I was a kid, as I've said. I've played football and many other sports, studied exercise physiology, and then trained people, including a lot of athletes. Olympians even.

I'm still amazed at how many young people in tremendous physical condition eat horribly. I did it, too, twenty-five years ago. Just watch high school and college athletes as they go from an intense practice and murderous drills straight to the fast-food drive-through. You'd think that to work so hard they'd have to eat and drink like champions. But they don't.

I know adults who have the same mentality. They'll say, well,

I burned 900 calories at the gym today, so I can go out and have three slices of pizza, or a pint of ice cream, or a bunch of tequila shooters, and it's okay.

But it's not. First of all, your body treats healthy, nutrient-dense calories differently than it does unhealthy, low-nutrient ones. Second, bad foods do a lot of bodily damage beyond the empty calories they contain. No amount of exercise can offset it.

And those young jocks in beautiful shape no matter what they eat? Imagine the condition they'd be in if they worked hard *and* ate well. I guarantee they would be even stronger and faster. Not only that, but they won't be young forever, and someday those bad habits will catch up with them. They'll be middle-aged and sedentary but still eating as though they were active nineteen-year-olds. The world is full of retired athletes who are now overweight, sickly, and falling apart. And as we've seen, the seeds of heart disease and cancer are often planted decades before they begin to blossom.

The links between physical activity and the five life forces are endless.

The more we move, the more oxygen we take in. And it doesn't have to be exercise per se—just daily, consistent movement. As we'll discuss later, oxygen is the fuel in every cell in our bodies. It's the spark that creates energy; it enhances our ability to recover and to repair our cells and tissues; it makes our blood flow more efficiently; and it makes our lungs more efficient. Researchers had some elderly women walk half an hour a day. That alone was enough to cut their risk of respiratory disease.

Exercise raises our body temperature, which causes us to sweat to cool off, which means we'll drink more water, which in turn improves everything else. Increased perspiration also helps our bodies get rid of toxins and acids.

Our detox systems benefit in other ways, too. The *Journal of the American Medical Association* published a study of three thousand women being treated for breast cancer; those with hormone-responsive tumors who walked briskly three to five hours a week reduced their risk of dying from the disease by half, compared to sedentary women.

When we exercise, our hearts work harder to pump more oxygen throughout the body, especially to the muscles, where it is most needed. This increases the capillary action; even the smallest blood vessels work to carry oxygen to our cells, which is good for our entire vascular system. The additional oxygen also increases the red blood cell count.

Exercise, by increasing the need for energy, steps up our natural metabolic processes, so more cellular debris needs to be cleared out. Activity increases the flow of lymphatic fluid, which helps to ward off disease.

When we get enough activity, we take something great and make it greater. If we increase our oxygen saturation, and our alkalinity, and our hydration, and our good nutrients, and our detox system, we are making ourselves nearly as healthy as possible. Then we begin to move, and we reach the highest level there is.

We should move a lot, but moderately for the most part—walking, doing things that require us to be on our feet and without shoes as much as possible. That works the foot muscles, which are often neglected, and it helps us improve our balance. It also just keeps us connected.

Quite a few studies lately have linked too much sitting with an increased risk of death. Scientists think being seated alters our metabolism. They aren't exactly sure why this is so, but it is. Stand whenever you can; you'll live longer.

But we must also engage in short periods of high-intensity activity. We should be explosive at those times. Sprinting—running or swimming or biking as fast as we can for short distances—is much better for us than the half-hour or longer jogging drudgery that I see people endure on treadmills. It's more fun, too. Even five minutes a day is enough, and it doesn't have to feel like working out. Chase your kids. Chase the dog. Jump up and down, climb a tree, hit some tennis balls against a wall, shadow-box a couple rounds. Do something that makes you pant and sweat.

These brief, high-intensity workouts give us great health benefits. They improve our metabolism, strength, quickness, and endurance, raise our natural growth hormone and testosterone levels, and improve our anti-aging factors.

We should also lift weights or take part in some form of resistance training, even just using body weight, but really challenging our muscle power to the max. Yes, women too! You can't get bulky from working out with weights. That myth has been passed around for far too long. No amount of weight lifting will give you a man's hormones. If we force our muscles to do more than they can comfortably handle, they respond by growing stronger. The lean tissue we build today will serve us for the rest of our lives. Nobody wants to be that old man or lady who has fallen and can't get up. A weight-training habit will guarantee that we'll always have the strength to perform the actions of everyday life. And our bones respond to stronger muscles by becoming denser and thicker, meaning less chance of osteoporosis.

Exercise builds our ability to balance, too—so we won't fall in the first place, and even if we do, our bones won't break, and we'll have the power and energy to hop right back up.

The old "pumping iron" mentality has gone away. Now we are aware that it's not necessarily how much we can lift but what we can do maintaining correct form—proper mechanics through a multiple-chained movement. What does that mean? Exercises such as kettle bell swings, burpees, Roman get-ups, body-weight movements like push-ups, pull-ups, squats, and lunges. We don't even need to "work out" in the traditional sense at all. We can just go outside and work in the garden or take a long walk every day.

Today, there are so many ways to get moving. If you don't have a gym handy, and there's nobody around to walk or bike with, you can fire up your DVD player and take a yoga class, or even "join" a high-intensity workout group in the privacy of your own home (like the P90X, 21-Day Fix or T25 programs offered by my colleagues at Beachbody).

In his book *The Blue Zones*, Dan Buettner visited places where people live long, active lives. His number-one lesson from the fit senior citizens he met was this: Move naturally. "They engage in regular, low-intensity physical activity, often as part of a daily work routine," he wrote.

Find what you enjoy in life and do it. Don't make it complicated; just move regularly, find the fun, play a lot, and you will enjoy long-term health benefits.

We need to honor the animal body, the being that wants to engage vigorously with the physical world. I train with my friend, the surf god Laird Hamilton, who said something wise while we were working out: "Do what you can't do, so you can do more of what you want to do."

Of course, that doesn't allow me to ride hundred-foot waves or other things only Laird can do in the water. But it means we should try new, hard things, movements that challenge our weaknesses. That's the only way we'll get stronger. The ability to respond, to play, to show up for life, are the reasons I challenge myself when I work out. I don't want to be limited by what my body can and can't do. I want a super life! Being able to play and move and do what I want is important to me.

But exercise shouldn't feel like drudgery. Make it a game. Compete, even if only against yourself. Do something where you feel you're going all out, the way kids do. Intensity is your friend. It stimulates growth-hormone production and makes our muscles strong. Don't just plod along on the treadmill, or hunch over the exercise bike, or load yourself into the leg press machine, or lie down on the bench and squeeze out presses, one after another. We need to go from one extreme to the other, from total rest to full-out crazy exertion—to make our movements a little unpredictable. A little chaotic but smart and controlled.

Like basketball—you jog, then suddenly you're down under the basket and a play explodes, and you are jumping and blocking and racing around in a tight little corner, and throwing and catching and shooting. And then the ball flies down the court and it happens all over again.

Moving at top speed, or lifting as much as we possibly can . . . it's not just healthy, it feels great. These are the moments when you realize that muscles can experience joy. Intense activity releases a flood of dopamine into our bloodstream, filling us with a kind of athletic ecstasy, even if we aren't exactly athletes. It's pure physical pleasure, and getting to that place is a wonderful thing. It's good for our souls. It reminds us what it means to be alive.

I believe that the deepest part of us is based in movement. All the internal systems that heal us and keep us safe from disease and inflammation work best when we are active. The mechanisms of healing, of optimal health, of brain activation and the production of neurochemicals like serotonin and dopamine, and proper sleep, and general outlook on life—they're all based in activity.

If we don't get the energy that comes from movement, we will seek it in caffeine or energy drinks or cigarettes. Chemical stimulation fries our adrenals and creates metabolic and hormone imbalances that can result in inflammation, poor sleep, digestive disorders, hypertension, and other unhealthy conditions in the body. If we don't get enough activity to make us tired at night, we will seek sleep in pills or alcohol.

We used to think that if you underwent surgery, you healed best by lying in bed. Or, if you hurt a body part, it got better if it was immobilized. Now we know the opposite is true. Moving is an important part of healing.

Studies have shown that we lose a significant percentage of our muscle mass if we don't use it. There's no such thing as maintaining fitness—either we get stronger or we get weaker.

But we don't need to beat ourselves into shape—that's not the way to do it. We shouldn't be stressing about it. I see people who go to the gym every day and yet their bodies never change and they don't seem to feel any better. You're supposed to feel great. That's the only thing that counts.

It's not about the perfect body or the perfect workout routine. You just need to show up for your own life. The sun came up today, and you're alive, and you have all the air and water and food you need. Now, what will you do with it?

I work out six times a week with a bunch of guys. The youngest are in their twenties, the oldest in their sixties. Three days we're in the gym, the other three we work out in a pool or in the ocean. We also surf together. We all have busy lives, but we make time first thing every day. We go pretty hard, but we have fun, too—we rib each other without mercy, and it gets salty. But we also cheer each other on and watch to make sure we're doing things right, so everybody gets strong and nobody gets hurt. Egos are left at the door. There's a lot of grunting and cursing and sweating and laughing. By now, it's become more than just exercise. We're buddies. We pay attention to what's going on in each other's lives.

As adults go, we do pretty well. But I've never seen anybody do it better than your average kid. Kids don't "work out"—they play. They move and push themselves and compete and wear themselves out, not because they think they should. Not because their doctors told them to. They do it because it's fun. That's the best reason for doing anything. Fun will motivate us when nothing else works, not even our own well-being.

The single best thing we can do to get in shape is to make it fun. The guys I work out with—we have fun.

# Simple To-Do List

- Get regular exercise. It acts on our bodies just as powerfully as the nutrients in our food or the medicines we take. You just can't be a healthy person if you don't move and challenge yourself physically.

- Find friends to play sports with, or exercise alongside. We can inspire each other and help one another to reach our potential better than we can alone.

- Bring true intensity to your workouts. Our bodies adapt to the stress and discomfort of exercise by making us stronger and more capable.

- If you are a woman who fears getting too muscular, relax. Women have less of the hormones that make bulky muscular growth possible.

- Maintain your strong muscles as you grow older.

- Don't work hard at the gym for an hour, only to sit behind a desk or on a sofa for the rest of the day. Move around a lot in your daily routine. The best physical activity doesn't take place in a gym or on a treadmill—we enjoy movement most when it's a part of our normal lives, walking and running around, jogging up and down the stairs, and playing with family, friends, and pets. Activity shouldn't be a special thing we do, it should be life itself.

# Life Force Number Three:
## Oxygenation

Want to know how important oxygen is? Hold your breath. We can live two months without food, two weeks without water, and maybe four minutes without oxygen. That tells us a lot.

Everybody knows we need oxygen to live, though most of us can't say exactly why. We breathe it into our lungs, where it enters the bloodstream—healthy plasma is at least 90 percent oxygen. It is taken up by the hemoglobin molecules and transported into cells everywhere. There, a protein combines the oxygen with other elements and turns it into water. The energy released in that transfer is what our cells use to fuel all their—our—functions.

Food is our other main source of energy, but without oxygen we can't get at the nutrients we eat. Without oxygen, nothing happens anywhere in our bodies. Its presence is required in just about every chemical reaction. It provides the spark of life. That's pretty important. Oxygen ignites our cells.

But this is the life force we take most for granted. We breathe involuntarily, and that's about all there is to say. One of those things that takes care of itself, right?

Wrong—plenty of us go through life with too little oxygen, and we pay a price. We can take steps to get more. But first it might help if we know how getting too little can harm us and impair the ability of the other four life forces to maintain our good health.

In 1931, Dr. Otto Warburg won the Nobel Prize in medicine for his discovery of the link between oxygen and cancer. It's worth hearing him explain it: "Cancer, above all other diseases, has countless secondary causes. But even for cancer, there is only one prime cause. Summarized in a few words, the prime cause of cancer is the replacement of the respiration of oxygen in normal body cells by a fermentation of sugar." (Cancer cells don't use oxygen for energy, depending on glucose instead.)

Warburg studied the metabolism of tumors and the respiration of cells, and that's how he saw the connection between low oxygen and cancer—or, said another way, the link between oxygen-rich tissues and good health. He was honored for that breakthrough in 1931, but today cancer is still our number-two killer. Just knowing about the link with oxygen deficiency hasn't been enough to prevent it.

By now the link between cancer and low oxygen has been repeatedly established. Recently, researchers from the University of Georgia published in the *Journal of Molecular Cell Biology* an analysis of samples of seven different types of cancer in the lab, finding that long-term lack of oxygen in cells caused the cancers to spread.

Obviously, this doesn't mean that if we just breathe deeper we won't get cancer. At the cellular level, oxygen content depends on many factors, which we'll discuss. Some are beyond our control. But if we do all we can to keep ourselves oxygen-rich and alkaline, those two life forces will combine to make our bodies more inhospitable to disease.

Dr. Arthur C. Guyton, author of the respected *Textbook of Medical Physiology*, put it like this: "All chronic pain, suffering and diseases are caused from a lack of oxygen at the cell level."

Wow. Consider the implications of that as we try to understand the importance of sufficient oxygen to our health. Not just *some* of the "pain, suffering and disease." *All*.

Oxygen can actually be medicine. Research reported in the *Journal of Critical Care* studied twenty-five patients admitted to a hospital with severe acute respiratory infections. Within six hours of undergoing oxygen therapy, more than 45 percent of them showed improvement. Oxygen therapy, the study concluded, "is an effective modality for early treatment of adults" with these infections. Doctors routinely prescribe hyperbaric chambers—exposure to 100 percent oxygen—for patients who need to repair damaged internal organs.

It's almost impossible to exaggerate the importance of oxygen to health. It has been studied more and for longer than any other element, especially its relation to well-being. Centuries ago, even the alchemists knew it was powerful.

Oxygen provides a perfect example of how interrelated the five life forces are. If our detox systems don't clear away toxins and carcinogens, they build up around and inside our cells, actually choking them. When that happens, cellular respiration is reduced—the flow of oxygen in and out is impaired. Another factor that lowers oxygenation of cells is poor blood circulation. And what causes that? Chiefly, improper diet—when we eat processed foods, unhealthy fats, and too much sugar, our red blood cells clump together and don't flow as they should.

Meanwhile, we may not be consuming enough of the essential fatty acids—contained in foods like walnuts, chia and flaxseed, algae, salmon, krill, and sardines—to maintain healthy cell walls. That's another cause of poor oxygen exchange.

Dr. Johanna Budwig, a German scientist, built on the work of Dr. Warburg by discovering that lipids—fats—are a powerful influence over cellular respiration, and therefore over oxygenation. We can take meaningful steps to prevent cancer, she said, by getting plenty of those essential fatty acids and none of the hydrogenated fats found mainly in—you guessed it—processed foods.

When we eat properly, our food can provide oxygen. When we drink plenty of water, it allows for greater oxygen exchange. If we foster a slightly alkaline inner environment by getting enough minerals in our diet, our cells will naturally be oxygen-rich. If our detox system is strong, it clears the cells of metabolic debris, helping to maintain a healthy cellular oxygen level. In turn, our oxygenated tissues support our immune system's efforts to keep us free of cancer and diseases caused by viruses and bacteria.

On the other hand, a lousy diet, too much protein, processed foods, too little water, excessive acidity, stress, and toxicity all add up to oxygen-poor cells and, eventually, an overwhelmed immune system.

## How Oxygen Can Harm

The main characteristic of oxygen is its power. It is potent rocket fuel. Fire can't burn without it. It is cleanser, sanitizer, deodorizer, purifier. Oxidation on metal is rust. Oxygen is what makes that apple core so ugly and brown after a little exposure.

In our bodies, oxygen has the power not only to create but also to destroy. We metabolize our food by mixing the nutrients with oxygen, helping to break it down, but the combination creates free radicals—atoms and molecules with odd numbers of electrons, which damage everything in their path. In an attempt to stabilize themselves with an even number of electrons, they steal an electron from every atom they crash into. The atoms and molecules they rob become free radicals, creating the same havoc wherever they go. Dr. Andrew Weil has compared it to a tornado tearing up everything in its path—a chain reaction of cellular damage that is associated with cancer and aging, among other badness. Oxygen is a double-edged sword.

We can combat this damage in a number of ways, mainly by consuming antioxidants, which neutralize free radicals and render them harmless. In "Life Force Number One: Nutrition," we discussed the importance of eating foods containing these cancer-fighting substances. Free radicals are a natural part of the turnover of life at the cellular level. As long as we eat fresh, whole food, we don't have to worry about the oxidative process.

Harm can also be done by too little oxygen, or hypoxia, which shows up everywhere. It narrows the vessels surrounding the brain and heart, reducing blood flow to those organs. It results in low sugar to the brain, which is a problem, since glucose is that organ's main nutrient. The biggest concern is that low-level oxygen deprivation can go unnoticed and, over time, cause chronic degeneration of the body and its various systems. As a study conducted at the University of Leeds, England, concludes, "There is a clear link between low oxygen levels in the brain and Alzheimer's disease."

Oxygen-poor cells lose some of their messaging capacity, which lessens their ability to adapt to changes in our internal environment and combat toxins we ingest. Too little oxygen has been found to trigger the sympathetic nervous system—our fight-or-flight response to threats. Even emotional and psychological stresses deplete oxygen, by releasing adrenaline and other related hormones. In a study done at the Osaka Institute of Social Medicine, Japan, mental stress was found to reduce the amount of oxygen that muscle cells were able to take up.

The symptoms of low cellular oxygen include fatigue, circulation problems, poor digestion, muscle aches and pain, dizziness, depression, memory loss, irrational behavior, irritability, acidic stomach, bronchial problems, and overall immune problems. Covers a lot of territory, doesn't it? These sound like the kind of "normal" complaints that a lot of supposedly healthy people have. Think maybe we'd feel healthier if we managed to get more oxygen into our tissues?

Dr. Leon Chaitow has studied hyperventilation, breathing so rapid and shallow that it delivers too little oxygen, which is more common in women than in men. Breathing improperly, he found, not deeply into the lower chest and stomach, can lead to chronic lower back pain and colon spasms, and even weaken the muscles of the core. The diaphragm can constrict and clamp down on the nerves and arterial blood flow and restrict digestive passage into the stomach.

Improper breathing is associated with a long list of ailments:

irritable bowels, allergies, headaches, and abnormal blood sugar. Even the cramps, sensitivity to pain, and irritability of premenstrual syndrome may be caused by too-shallow breathing, triggered by monthly hormonal changes.

To a large degree, low oxygen is due to our unhealthy behaviors, mostly our eating and drinking habits. But some of it can be blamed on the planet's bad health, too.

Prior to the Industrial Revolution, the air contained around 32 percent oxygen. Today, in the world's major cities, it's 15 percent—half as much. Our need for oxygen hasn't decreased. In fact, due to all the toxins we must now neutralize, we need more oxygen than ever, and get less. Ervin Laszlo, a UN adviser and professor of philosophy and systems sciences, writes: "At these levels it is difficult for people to get sufficient oxygen to maintain bodily health: it takes a proper intake of oxygen to keep body cells and organs, and the entire immune system, functioning at full efficiency. At the levels we have reached today cancers and other degenerative diseases are likely to develop. And at 6 to 7 percent life can no longer be sustained."

The planet itself contains less oxygen than it once did, and, like us, it struggles to maintain its health as a result. Count up the square miles of rain forest vegetation that disappear every year, and bear in mind that green plants are 40 percent oxygen, which they release into the atmosphere. It's not just the air. A huge amount of our oxygen is created and released by the plankton and phytoplankton, some of the smallest and oldest green plant life in the oceans. As the seas become warmer and more polluted, the oxygen level drops, and plant life suffers. We do, too. Everywhere on the planet, oxygen equals life.

## Keeping Oxygenated

So what can we do to keep our own oxygen healthy? The answers lie largely in the other life forces.

First, we can do it through diet. Raw vegetables, fruits, nuts, and seeds are best. Raw and fresh because oxygen is contained there. Leafy greens especially—plants with high chlorophyll content, like kale, chard, spirulina, and chlorella. Raw, fresh food equals higher oxygen! Cooking speeds up the oxidation of anything we eat. Foods that don't contribute oxygen—which include animal products, processed foods, and sugar—deplete it instead. As with everything else, nutrition is key.

Drinking enough high-quality water is next. When water flows in nature, in lakes or streams, it is aerated by the movement, making the oxygen it contains more stable and available to the body. As we discussed in "Life Force Number Two: Hydration," few of us drink daily from unpolluted springs, so we need to make a little effort to get clean water, structured by mineral content and movement.

As Dr. Warburg found, there is a close tie between oxygen and healthy cellular alkalinity. We can help our bodies to keep us slightly alkaline through diet and by avoiding the things—certain foods and drinks, toxins, even negative emotions—that acidify us. "Life Force Number Four: Alkalization" discusses this in detail.

Doing all we can to keep our detox strong also helps our tissues stay oxygen-rich. It rids our cells of junk, natural and otherwise, that depresses the tissues' ability to hold oxygen. If our kidneys can't get rid of toxins, they stay in the bloodstream, and that also decreases the amount of oxygen our blood is able to carry. If we adopt the habits that keep external poisons to a minimum—I mean pollution, household toxins, everyday irritants—we only help. I'll talk more about detoxification in "Life Force Number Five: Detoxification."

Even keeping plants around us is beneficial for maintaining healthy levels of oxygen in our systems. Plants are very effective air purifiers, nature's most efficient indoor air cleaners, removing pollutants such as formaldehyde, benzene, trichloroethylene, even dust. Studies have shown that hospital patients who have plants in their rooms recover more quickly.

Finally, we can just breathe better. More.

Yogis and monks have many reasons to meditate, but what unites them all is the breath. Not only is breathing meditative and good for calming stress, but it improves brain and immune system function, cleanses the body, and purifies our minds. A simple technique I use in the morning is the 5-5-5-5 method: Inhale slowly on a count of five, then hold the breath for five seconds, exhale to a count of five, and finally count to five with no breathing at all and nothing in your lungs. I do this for about fifteen minutes every day.

Most of us don't fill our lungs to capacity when we inhale; thus, we don't take in all the oxygen we're capable of getting. There are a number of ways to fix this.

One is just to become more mindful of our breathing. Typically, we take too-shallow breaths—usually from stress—filling only the top part of our lungs. For most normal activity, that's all the air we need—unfortunately. We need to focus on filling our lungs, and then fully expelling their contents, which include harmful gases.

If we're not getting regular physical activity, we won't need to breathe very deeply. That's yet another good argument for exercise—the habits we pick up there may carry over into the rest of our lives. If we begin breathing more when we move, our bodies may remember the pleasant sensation.

That's a reason we need to experience intensity when we exercise. If our hearts pound and we pant like crazy, we're taking in all the oxygen we can. My friends and I do a pool workout using dumbbells—we perform Navy Seal–type exercises that make us work underwater while holding our breath, then race to the surface to gulp air. It's intense, but when we finish it's the best feeling ever.

*Aerobics* is the old-fashioned term for exercise that makes us breathe hard. Nowadays people tend to do it mainly because it helps us lose weight and keep it off. But the physiological benefits go way beyond that. It's no coincidence that athletes have a greater lung capacity than nonathletes, though their lungs are no bigger.

Higher oxygen intake is also closely associated with improved heart health. Anything that makes us breathe deeply is good.

Muscles are nice, but it's even better to exercise for a strong heart and lungs.

Simply reminding ourselves to breathe deeper can make a difference. That's a benefit of yoga, where breath control is so important. And I highly recommend some form of meditation, some place in your life where you can stop, consciously breathe, and reflect.

As a reminder, every time I eat, I use it as a stop time, giving thanks to my food and breathing through my nose, slowing my body, preparing to receive the food by shifting to a calm, parasympathetic state.

I love to surf. It teaches us the power of breath, how to cherish it, the life or death importance of oxygen. Every time I get held under by a wave, I am humbled by the power of this life force.

When we use our bodies to the maximum, the message we are sent is constant: *Breathe.* That's a great reminder of the power and importance of this life force.

# Simple To-Do List ✓

- Do everything possible to get lots of oxygen into your body. Don't just inhale it—make sure to get oxygen from the foods you eat, like fresh fruit and vegetables. The symptoms of too little oxygen in our cells show up everywhere, from fatigue to immunity problems to Alzheimer's disease.

- Breathe consciously. That means inhaling deeply, to fill your lungs, and then empty them completely. Too many people breathe shallowly. Breathing deeply through the nose is also a great stress reliever, immediately calming the body, and it's safer and cheaper than Valium.

- Go outdoors. The concentration of oxygen in the air is higher outdoors than indoors, so spend more time surrounded by trees and grass, which make the air cleaner and richer. Remember, oxygen is medicine.

- Inhale properly through your nose, which filters out the dirt, pollution, and other weirdness that would otherwise go straight into the lungs.

- Get some exercise every day. Physical activity requires you to inhale and exhale deeply and in a controlled way, thereby encouraging good breathing habits.

- Where your breath goes, you go. If it is short and rapid, the body will be stressed and tight. When it is deep and full, the body is loose and relaxed.

# My Life as a Superfood Hunter

It all started pretty much by accident. It was the 1990s, and power bars were in style—a good idea, making quick hits of energy and nutrition as convenient and portable as a candy bar. The problem was that they tasted horrible and contained lots of bad ingredients—refined sugars and processed grains and chemical additives.

So I decided I'd make my own at home. I'd take some almond butter and coconut and seeds and nuts and dried fruit, a little protein powder, some spirulina, everything raw and natural, and mix it together, then shape it into bars. And I'd put them into a container and take them with me wherever I went, like to the gym or the beach. People liked them, so I kept experimenting with new and better ingredients—researching, exploring, traveling, testing, testing, and more testing, for years.

Then, my father died and left me a little money. I decided I'd use it to start a company that would seriously search everywhere for the best-quality, most nutrient-dense foods—power foods, medicinal plants, or superfoods, we'd call them today—and put them into formulas people could drink, or elixirs, or simply use as raw ingredients. I just wanted to find new things, the cleanest and most powerful, and get them out into the world.

If I heard about something special that grew in the Himalayas, for instance, now I could jump on a plane and go there to see for myself. I didn't want to just buy commercially processed versions of things or rely on someone else finding my products for me. By then I was a veteran control freak when it came to what I put in my body. You can't assume that your food doesn't contain chemicals, GMOs, or other weird ingredients. You would be amazed at how careless and blissfully ignorant some processors and manufacturers are about the plants that go into their products.

My motto was: Don't destroy this perfection! I was determined to care for the plant from the soil through the growth and drying and processing to keep intact as much of its extraordinary power as possible, all the vitamins, minerals, and healing properties that support our bodies. Nature alone creates perfect food to help us thrive; anything made in a lab always comes with an unwelcome side effect or two, or twenty. I wanted to go into the wild and to the farms where food grew, to see it in the dirt and talk to the farmer about what it did and why and how people there used it. That's how I really enjoy learning. I have a BA and a master's degree, but all that education pales in comparison to this type of passionately experiential adventure.

Along the way I met an amazing guy, Miguel Beruman, who had been working at a vitamin store here in Malibu. He and I were in tune with each other in how we wanted to find the best foods in a sustainable way that was also fair to the people we got them from. Miguel was wickedly smart and educated in the science of natural health and herbs. I hired him to help me figure out how to turn those superfoods into a product that we could manufacture and sell to benefit people. Miguel now lives in Argentina, which helps to keep us in contact with growers and researchers in Latin America and around the world. The fact that he speaks several languages and comes from generations of indigenous Mexican/ Native American healers is also a huge asset.

Then I was introduced to Isabelle and Carl Daikeler, the couple behind the company called Beachbody. I didn't have a TV at the time, so I had no idea about their hugely successful exercise empire, which includes programs like P90X, Insanity, T25, Turbo Fire, Brazilian Butt Lift, and more. Isabelle met Miguel at the vitamin store, and she mentioned that the company of her boyfriend at the time, now her husband, was working on an idea for a supplement shake. He steered her to me, and changed the trajectory of my life. Isabelle and Carl wanted to create a high-end, no-compromises superfood meal replacement shake like nothing that existed at that time—something that even I, a maniac for pure, healthy ingredients, would drink. They wanted me to develop it, and they would market it. Two years of hard work later, the formula was ready to go. In 2008, we unleashed Shakeology. Today, hundreds of thousands of people benefit from it every day.

Superfood hunting has taken me all over the world. I make three or four extended trips a year, one region at a time. Sometimes I'll have a contact in an area; sometimes I just pick a place based on a little information and a gut feeling. I read lots of scientific articles and meet academic and clinical researchers who devote their lives to the study of health. I meet and work with indigenous farmers all over the world, and Third World shamans and healers who use herbs and plants to make people healthier.

From the start, this was the way I decided it had to be structured. Instead of finding a commercial supplier who would sell me the ingredients in bulk, I went directly to the source. I wanted to know everything about the plants first—how they grew and where, who grew them and harvested them. It was my version of fair trade before I knew what fair trade was. I wanted to be sure everybody was getting a good deal. I knew that if the ingredients had come through a processor or a wholesaler, the people who grew it were probably getting screwed. I wanted to help improve the lives of the people who provided us with the foods; if their lives were better, they would make better business partners. I wanted to be part of the deal. If you don't experience the ride on the yak to reach the fields of the product you want, you don't really know the product. You can buy palm oil from lots of sources, but most of it involves killing off orangutans by stripping clean their habitats. I don't want it, if that's what it involves. You can get palm oil without harming animals or people.

Every time I travel to find new foods, I learn unexpected things—about new herbs, or new uses for them that I'd never imagined before. Sometimes the scientists tell me something I didn't know, and I can contact a shaman and ask his opinion. Sometimes it's the other way around.

My main talent is that I show up. I'm addicted to action. Once I heard something good about the moringa tree, which grows in Senegal, among other places. I had a contact there, someone I barely knew—we had talked just once—but I had a good feeling about him, and I had already done some research into the tree and the place, so I went. It was worth the trip—the moringa leaves have seven times the amount of vitamin C in oranges, four times the calcium and double the protein in milk, four times the vitamin A in carrots, and three times the potassium in bananas. They contain many powerful antioxidants, too.

Moringa is easy to grow in subtropical regions, but hard to process, so all over the developing world people cultivate it and eat the leaves fresh and in cooking. In places where no one can afford fancy pharmaceuticals, moringa trees keep people healthy. One nickname for it is "the vitamin tree," and in Senegal they call it "the never-die tree" for its healing powers.

We do our best to retain its goodness by processing it intelligently and with care. We wash it and dry it in the shade as soon as it's picked, to retain the nutrients and antioxidants, and then pulverize it as soon as we can. It is imperative to know the essential nature of each food to understand how best to process it. There's no such thing as one type of processing for all. Doing it our way is a lot of work, and it costs more. But you have to do what's right to maintain the innate nutrition of the food. If you care about quality, there is no other way.

But before anything else can happen, we first have to find a fair way to structure the market. Most of the time the negotiations happen around a campfire in the village, just you and the tribal leaders. Sometimes they're glad to hear you're interested, sometimes it doesn't work out. You have to get a feel for how they operate and how they think about the plant before you can figure out how to get it. I still work with the rural communities of this African nation to create fair trade, stimulate economy, and grow and process the best moringa in the world.

Baobob is another great find from West Africa. It grows in the wild, and the people consider the tree sacred—it carries the spirit of those who have passed on, they believe. It also produces an amazing fruit with tons of nutrients. Because it's not farmed, you need the local people to go into the woods and collect it for you.

To set up a steady supply, I had to negotiate deals with three different villages. While we talked, I asked them about their drinking water supply, which is often a problem in poor regions of the world, and they said they could use some help with that. So I got them filters through RainCatcher.org, an international group I'm involved with, and they felt comfortable enough to do business. When the intention is not just to take but to support a trade partner, then you truly have a win-win situation and a fair exchange.

A day like that is incredible because you've changed people's lives by getting them fresh water, and you've also given them an economic boost. They don't need a lot of money, they don't need a lot of things, but you've helped them with some life-sustaining changes, and they've helped you. And together you're bringing a healthy food to people all over the world. But to get to that point, to those few hours with the tribes, you spend hundreds of hours flying and riding along unpaved roads, and it takes years to set up sometimes. And that's the only way to do it. To this day I am involved directly in the development of indigenous African superfoods like moringa and others, all of which began when I had a good feeling and did something about it.

I go to India and people ask, Hey, how was the Taj Mahal? and I say I missed it because I was in a car for twenty-five hours so I could spend an hour on some guy's farm. I was there to find plants in the natural environment. I don't want to deal with brokers or processors, I want to see the stuff growing, I want to learn all about it and how it fits in with the culture that makes it possible. I'm glad that these farmers and our team can help create a healthier world in a responsible way—it's better than cutting down the trees or selling the land to some mining company. But mostly I do it for the absolute awe of getting my mind blown by new food, new culture, and extraordinary people.

I've had some interesting experiences with the non-plant world, too.

I spent a few days in the rain forest in northeastern Australia, among the wild boars and poisonous snakes, looking at kakadu plum, jackfruit, dragonfruit, cacao, and other superfoods that grow there. For a change, I was staying in a pretty nice hotel. One evening I was walking down a path toward my room, not really paying attention, when I looked up and saw a huge Komodo dragon blocking my way. He was as big as I was and probably weighed the same, too. I wasn't even sure what it was—I thought at first it was a weird-looking alligator. Only later did I find out that a Komodo dragon's bite can easily kill a human. We stared at each other for a moment, and then he turned and we both walked away. I figured I could come back later when he'd moved on.

Just another day at the office. My passion has become my business, and now it's all I do. You start out asking things like "What does my body need that it's not getting?" And the questions never stop. The more I learn, the more I want to know.

# Which Ones Are Right for You?

Of course, people are always asking me which superfoods they should be eating. It comes with the territory.

Unfortunately, the answer is never that simple.

First, we need to understand the proper uses of superfoods. They are a way of bridging a gap. They're not cure-alls. They should fit in somewhere between our normal food intake and our nutritional supplements and medicines. Nobody's going to start the day with a big bowl of dried goji berries. (Well, OK, maybe a few of us!) But we can't eat doughnuts and sugary cereal for breakfast and then hope to fix everything by loading up at the superfood counter.

These potent substances should be a regular part of our diet. But first we need to understand their uses and apply them according to our needs.

For example, we all need to consume vitamin C. Once, our bodies were able to manufacture it on their own, but we lost the ability because it was so abundant in the plants we ate. Today, however, few of us get enough from our food.

Lots of people rely on a typical store-bought supplement, a pill or capsule that isolates ascorbic acid. But there are superfoods that contain incredibly high levels of the vitamin, and in a form that is immediately accessible to our bodies. Camu camu is a reddish-purple cherry-like fruit that grows in the Amazon rain forest. It is one of the most potent natural fruit sources of the vitamin; typically, its powder contains 10 to 20 percent naturally occurring vitamin C. And it's more effective than ascorbic acid alone.

As I mentioned, the leaves of the moringa tree have seven times as much Vitamin C as an orange, plus high levels of antioxidants and other nutrients. And there are many other such sources of vitamin C, which is so critically important to our ability to defend ourselves from disease. This is the purpose of superfoods—to provide the high-powered nutrient density that we no longer get from our usual meals.

In "Life Force Number Four: Alkalization," we'll discuss the importance of maintaining a slightly alkaline internal environment, and the ways that proper nutrition can help us attain that goal. There are also superfoods that alkalize us, as well as providing many powerful minerals and electrolytes in a form that is receptive to the body, foods such as chlorella, spirulina, blue-green algae, and marine phytoplankton. You don't fix yourself a big plate of any of these. But they exist in stable, carefully dried powders, or in elixirs that can be added to smoothies or shakes.

Science is still discovering all the ways that chronic inflammation harms our tissues and shortens our lives. Turmeric has been used for thousands of years as an effective anti-inflammatory that also has healing powers. I make a paste by mixing it with raw honey and almond or coconut milk, and eat a couple tablespoons every day. I just mix it in with whatever I happen to be eating. Turmeric is such a strong detoxifier that eating too much can create excessive heat and dryness in our liver tissue. For that reason it has to be balanced out with the honey, or licorice or cardamom. Otherwise, it's a little intense over a very long period of time. It is a good rule to cycle foods by taking a break from some and adding new ones. This doesn't have to be complicated. You can simply eat a lot of red foods for a while, then switch to yellow or purple.

Pineapple may not seem like a power food, but the enzyme it contains, bromalin, is an anti-inflammatory. Other systemic enzymes commonly available in health food stores, such as papain and protease, are also extremely effective.

When we exercise, we actually cause microscopic tears in the muscle, which create inflammation. In order to counter that and speed recovery, I am a big fan of fresh or freshly frozen coconut water or coconut milk, to regain necessary sugars as well as electrolyte minerals. I'll throw in some soaked chia seeds for fats and proteins, or plant proteins like pea, brown rice, and moringa for alkalizing the tissues and restoring the amino acids.

The harmful effects of stress—physical, emotional, environmental—come up again and again in this book. Our bodies respond to it by releasing the hormone cortisol, which can be damaging in the long term. We can provide a constant counterbalance to stress by eating ginseng, rhodiola, tongkat ali, astragalus, ashwagandha, and holy basil. Good versions of these can be found in pills and capsules as well as in powder form or as extracts.

Antidepressants are among the most commonly prescribed drugs today, even though science has proven how strongly nutrition influences our mental and emotional states. Having struggled with attention-deficit problems as a kid, and then overcome them as an adult and helped many others, I really understand the connection between how our brains function and what we eat and drink.

The first thing we need to do to support our brains is eliminate refined sugars and many of the refined grains and processed foods and increase water intake. But we can assist our neurotransmitters with foods like cacao and blue-green algae, both of which contain huge natural concentrations of phenylethylamine, which increases our output of dopamine, the feel-good chemical. The compounds in these superfoods go after the same neurotransmitter receptors as dopamine does, with no side effects and only sustainable, healthy balance and benefits. How great is that?

Chronic fatigue is usually due to behaviors that overstimulate the adrenal glands. We often respond by drinking stimulants such as coffee, soda, and energy drinks, which only makes it worse. The so-called adaptogenic herbs balance, support, and restore the body and increase our resistance to stress. Astragalus, tonkat ali, ginseng, cordyceps mushrooms, maca, rhodiola, and ashwagandha will help. So will eating goji berries or drinking green tea.

To make sure you're getting enough vitamin D, you can try getting more sunlight. That is the best way to get this very important nutrient. Remember, though, that sunblock prevents the healthy rays of the sun from getting in. So we need to go without it, while still taking care not to burn. Depending on where you live, however, or how much time you spend outdoors, you may need to supplement it.

There are plenty of vitamin D pills on the market, and they may be necessary during the winter months. Phytoplankton also contains vitamin D. Mushrooms that have been exposed to ultraviolet light will provide vitamin D, but this doesn't include many mushrooms you'll find in stores. You can either buy them and expose them to UV light—which may be more work than you bargain for— or find mushroom-based supplements that come from varieties that have been exposed to the light. The information is usually found on the labels.

Omega-3 fats are extremely important to good health. Lots of people supplement theirs through fish oil, but we have to ask ourselves: What are those fish eating? It's safer and healthier to get omega-3s from freshly ground flaxseed (you can use a coffee-bean grinder), chia seed, or an algae-based supplement. You can also get them from the oil of sacha inchi, an amazing plant from the Peruvian Amazon.

Recently I read a study that found a significant reduction in breast cancer in women who ate one teaspoon of freshly ground flaxseed daily. It also helped women who experience breast pain during menstruation. Such a small amount of powdered seed, and yet it can make such a big difference. That's what a superfood can do.

The fact that so many superfoods come in powder form makes smoothies and shakes an important part of a healthy diet. Adding these substances to some berries and greens and water or juice or a cultured dairy product like yogurt or kefir makes them easy to consume. So maybe you'll need a good blender to really take advantage of my advice.

As with supplements, it's hard to know which specific products are worthy and which don't really deliver what they promise. There's no way to tell what you're getting, short of using DNA-fingerprint-type technology. That's what we use at Shakeology to verify our raw materials, but that's not going to help you. The only advice I can offer is to find good, ethical companies that insist on supplying pure, unadulterated products. Later in this book I've provided a guide to good sources of superfoods—companies that sell clean, healthy substances. Start there.

# Simple To-Do List

- Eat plenty of nutrient-dense superfoods that provide high levels of biologically beneficial compounds to help the body heal and thrive.

- When possible, eat food rather than some vitamin or mineral produced in a lab and turned into a pill for nutrients. It's better to get vitamin C from, say, powdered moringa tree leaves or camu camu. This is the beauty of superfoods—they give pure, high-octane, biologically assimilative nutrition without the junk.

- Buy superfoods only from companies that respect the food itself, the farmer, the soil, and the source. If you read enough labels on enough brands, you'll begin to discern which firms really try to offer a clean, healthy, ethically sourced product from those that treat superfood as just another item on a store shelf.

- Enjoy superfoods the way you do everything else you eat—not as some kind of weird additive to your diet. Goji berries are delicious. We eat them the way some people snack on popcorn or M&Ms, but they happen to provide medicine to your body.

# Life Force Number Four: Alkalization

If you made it through junior high school science, you've probably met up with these two letters together before: pH.

They refer to the potential power of the hydrogen contained in any given substance. Maybe litmus paper was involved, showing you and the other kids how to test for pH. The number shows the balance of acidity to its opposite, alkalinity, in whatever it is we're measuring. More hydrogen means more acidic means lower pH number.

We all understand acid—it's corrosive, burning, it breaks things down. But this alkalization concept is hard to picture. Unlike nutrition, hydration, or oxygenation, we don't really get a mental image on this one.

Maybe that's why alkalization is the least understood of the five life forces. Ask even a health-conscious person, "How's your alkaline-acid balance?" and you'll get a blank stare back. Ask your physician, and the result will possibly be the same.

Our bodies understand all this acid-alkaline stuff very well, even if we don't. The balance between the two is essential to our health. But it's not a static condition—it ebbs and flows as the body and its environment change. This is one of the many instances where the body knows how to do things that the conscious mind could never manage.

As we go, keep this in mind: Every aspect of our health depends on us maintaining the proper internal alkaline-acid environment. And for a number of reasons, that's more challenging than it used to be.

# Why Too Much Acidity Harms Us

The most important thing to remember is that we should be, overall, slightly alkaline.

This is for a number of reasons. The proteins in our bodies function properly only at very specific pH levels, a little more alkaline than acidic. Our enzymes, which are specialized proteins, are sensitive to acidity, too. An overly acidic environment suppresses enzymatic action, which—as we talked about in "Life Force Number One: Nutrition"—negatively affects everything in our bodies, everywhere, at every level. It impairs our ability to metabolize what we eat, which in turn makes us even more acidic, creating an unhealthy cascade.

All our tissues and membranes become irritated and inflamed when they're acidified. They actually look and feel different—hardened, diseased.

Alkalinity, by contrast, is a soothing influence on our bodies. When we are alkaline, our tissues hold more oxygen, which supports all the cellular functions, including our ability to rid ourselves of toxins, harmful microbes, and metabolic debris.

We've already discussed Dr. Otto Warburg, the German scientist who won the 1931 Nobel Prize in medicine for his discovery of the link between low oxygen and cancer. He found that cancer cells are always highly acidic—the disease actually acidifies us. Science is still trying to fully understand the links between cancer and acidity, but there's no doubt they exist. So you can see how having too much acid in our bodies might not be such a great thing.

The scale that measures pH goes from 0 to 14. Neutral—neither acidic nor alkaline—is 7.0, right in the middle. But the scale is logarithmic, not arithmetic, an important difference. It means that each full point equals not one more or less than the point next to it, but ten times more or less. So, a substance with a pH of 5 is ten times more acidic than one with a pH of 6, and one hundred times more acidic than one with a pH of 7, and one thousand times more acidic than one with a pH of 8.

Here's a good example. Distilled water's pH is 7.0. Coca-Cola's is around 2.5. This means that a sugary, carbonated Coke is fifty thousand times more acidifying than pure water. Imagine what the acid in those sodas is doing to our insides. Not a pretty thought, is it?

Optimal body pH varies from one kind of tissue or fluid to another. For example, blood must have a pH between 7.35 and 7.45. That's slightly alkaline. If blood pH were to go below 6.8 or above 7.8, all our cells would stop functioning and we'd quickly die. (Don't worry—it won't happen.) Normal pH of the lungs is about the same. Normal eye pH is slightly more acidic, between 7.0 and 7.3. Stomach pH has to be way down at 2.0 to 3.0, because it requires lots of acid to do its digestive work of liquefying food. That's especially true if we've eaten meat, which requires stomach pH of about 0.8 to properly break down animal protein into amino acids.

Nearly every biochemical or electrical event that takes place inside us—energy creation, metabolism, oxidation, immune system response—has an acidifying effect. But when the balance does change, even a little, our bodies automatically adjust pH levels back to where they should be. That ability is more proof of how critical alkalinity is to our survival.

## How We Do It

Our lungs are part of the alkalizing mechanism. Every time we exhale, we excrete acids in the carbon dioxide. This is part of normal cellular metabolism. Whenever it's necessary to lower acidity, our bodies simply increase our breathing rate a little. We never even notice.

Our skin also plays a role. Our bodies push acids to the surface, where they can be released in sweat through the pores. (You may have noticed that it's almost always excess acidity we're dealing with, rarely alkalinity, for reasons I'll explain later.) If we need to get rid of acid, our sweat becomes more acidic. Again, we have no clue this is going on. In fact, our skin is always slightly acidic, which keeps it cohesive and also kills bacteria.

But it's our kidneys, those workhorses, that regulate overall blood composition and keep our acid-alkaline balance right. They do this by sensing our blood pH and then filtering out hydrogen ions if we're too acidic (or bicarbonate, when we're too alkaline). From there, the acids are excreted from our bodies through the normal exits, the colon and bladder.

Our kidneys, however, have a built-in limitation. They can't speed up the rate at which they filter blood, even if their workload increases, so they can process only so much at a time. When they are hit with more than they can handle, the unwanted substances just circulate in our bloodstream until the kidneys get around to dealing with them. This poses hazards of its own, of course, as the toxins or acids travel over and over through our vessels, damaging us on every pass.

We become acidic for several reasons. Perhaps our immune systems aren't working properly, and we're not ridding ourselves of toxins or harmful bacteria as we should. Or perhaps we're underhydrated, so we're not flushing metabolic debris and other normal cellular residue. A study published in the *European Journal of Clinical Nutrition* found that even mild dehydration can cause changes in the kidneys, including renal acidosis—dangerously high levels of acidity in the kidneys.

If our tissues aren't getting enough oxygen, we may become more acidic. Even emotional turmoil plays a part, releasing stress hormones that acidify us. Unhealthy relationships and negative self-image create mental patterns that affect us as surely as any physical factors. Where the mind goes, we go.

The other main culprit is diet. Food either alkalizes or acidifies our internal environment. The foods we eat, once we metabolize them, leave behind an actual ash, either acidic or alkaline. As an article titled "Examining the Relationship between Diet-Induced Acidosis and Cancer," published in the journal *Nutrition & Metabolism*, stated, "Acidogenic (acid forming) diets, which are typically high in animal protein and salt and low in fruits and vegetables, can lead to a sub-clinical or low-grade state of metabolic acidosis." And according to "Origins and Evolution of the Western Diet: Health Implications for the 21st Century," in the *American Journal of Clinical Nutrition*, "Healthy adults consuming the standard U.S. diet sustain a chronic, low-grade pathogenic metabolic acidosis that worsens with age as kidney function declines."

For the most part, the foods we should be eating lots of—fresh leafy greens, brightly colored vegetables, avocados, almonds, fresh cold-pressed oils such as olive oil—are alkalizing. Raw vegetables are very alkalizing. Fresh lemons and limes, though they are themselves acidic, also have an alkalizing effect on our bodies.

Likewise, the foods we should either avoid completely or eat in moderation—added refined sugars, meat, fish, and other animal foods and animal fats, processed foods, refined grains, coffee additives, flavoring agents, dyes—are all very acidifying, yet another problem associated with the standard American diet.

Now, there are quite a few exceptions to these rules. Some healthy foods, such as most beans, including lentils and peanuts, are slightly acidifying. All kinds of protein (even vegetable protein) and whole grains also acidify us mildly. So do many nuts and seeds. There are even some necessary, beneficial minerals that acidify us, such as sulfur, iodine, and phosphorus.

But plant-based foods contain so-called weak acids, which our bodies neutralize easily, mainly through respiration. In addition, alkalizing minerals such as potassium, which help cancel out any acidification, usually accompany plant protein.

Animal protein, on the other hand, contains the so-called strong acids such as uric, sulfuric, and phosphoric acid, which are not so easy to process. Uric acid, which crystallizes and collects in the joints, is the cause of gout, a painful disease that once struck only the few who could afford to eat meat often.

Our kidneys can handle the strong acids over time only with a little help from the liver, which does its part by secreting a highly alkaline substance, ammonia. This does a great deal to neutralize acids, but it's not so good for our tissues, and too much of it can cause blisters on the liver, cirrhosis, and acidosis in the long run.

How about water? When still, it's alkalizing, but any drink that fizzes is acidifying because of the carbonic acid that makes the bubbles—hence the term *carbonated*. The sugar in drinks just increases this effect. A study published in the *Korean Journal of Critical Care Medicine* bears this out, finding that subjects with the highest blood sugar levels had "significantly higher" metabolic acidosis: "These findings suggest that blood glucose level affects acid-base balance."

Oxygen? Alkalizing. Oxygen and alkalinity go hand in hand even at the cellular level. An alkaline environment is always oxygen-rich, and vice versa.

Exercise? It's neither acidic nor alkaline, but its effects can have a beneficial, alkalizing influence. However, too little exercise, or too much, can be acidifying. A strenuous workout will create lactic acid, which is then metabolized and neutralized by respiration. The lactic acid causes the burn and the soreness. That's acidity. But it's perfectly normal—that's how our bodies are meant to work. Too little exercise is unhealthy in every way.

Too little sleep and too much worry can stress our cells and be acidifying, too. If you're going to eat that big, juicy steak, just do it; agonizing over it will only make it worse. This is a key point. We all eat unhealthy things sometimes, and then make ourselves suffer mentally for doing it. When we consume that entire stack of Oreo cookies, then beat ourselves up over it, the ill effects are compounded by our shame, creating even more acidification.

Nicotine and caffeine are acidifying. So is alcohol. So is that popular herbal inebriator, marijuana, contrary to what you may have hoped. Other recreational drugs acidify us, too, and likewise prescription and over-the-counter medicines are even worse. You may begin to see a pattern here.

Life itself is acidifying, at least nowadays. This is why, as I said earlier, our bodies typically have to work to keep us slightly alkaline. Think of all the chemicals we're exposed to, all the pollutants and toxins and irritants, from the deadly to the merely irritating—in the air we breathe, the fabrics we wear, the cleaning chemicals that touch everything that touches us. We have no idea what we take in from the environment, but it all contributes to the overall acidity of life.

A good example is something called propylene glycol, an industrial chemical used in food preservatives and artificial flavorings for everything from toothpaste and shampoo to tobacco and pharmaceuticals. It's practically everywhere you look. According to the Centers for Disease Control, it is "oxidatively converted to lactic and pyruvic acids which, if present in sufficient amounts, contribute to a metabolic acidosis."

Exhaust gases emitted by gasoline, diesel fuel, natural gas, fuel oil, and coal have been found to affect the lungs, leading to breathing problems and something called respiratory acidosis—excessively acidic lung tissue.

Finally, look at what's happening to the oceans. As pollution starves them of oxygen, the seas become more acidic, choking the beneficial algae and other plant life found there. The same thing takes place inside our bodies. That's why I say that staying alkaline today is tougher than ever.

Here's a common way we experience the effects of too much acidity: acid reflux, that burning in the throat. People just swallow some Tums or Rolaids and try to live with it. That's not such a good idea. Our digestive tract is trying to tell us something—we're eating too much acidifying food. Instead of changing our diet, we take an acid neutralizer (both those products are mainly calcium, the alkalizing mineral). It goes right into our stomachs, which is where we actually need high levels of proper acidity, to digest our food. And once again our bad habits make it difficult for our bodies to do what they are meant to do.

# The Danger of Chronic Acidification

Keep in mind, however, that we need a certain level of acidity to live. We're not going for total abstinence here. Acid isn't a toxin or a harmful substance. We're just trying to strike a balance, which is sometimes the most challenging thing of all.

As I mentioned earlier, our blood alkaline-acid balance is of life-or-death importance. Luckily, our bodies won't allow that pH level to veer into the danger zone, even if our diet and habits are less than ideal. But to maintain that proper pH level, our bodies sometimes have to take measures that actually cause us harm over time.

Here's what happens if our acidity begins to outpace our bodies' ability to balance it:

Nothing.

Nothing we notice, at least at first.

That's because even when our kidneys can't properly adjust the acid-alkaline balance, there's a backup system ready to go.

Calcium, sodium, magnesium, and other minerals we contain are highly alkaline. If we become too acidic, we simply withdraw some minerals and send them where they are needed to buffer the acids. If our kidneys detect that our blood pH has lowered, they will automatically find the minerals needed to fix it. The alkaline chemically combines with the acid to produce a neutral salt, which is then safely eliminated. Yet another miracle going on in there without us even knowing. Excess acidification prompts an immediate alkalizing response.

But if our bodies are so good at maintaining the acid-alkaline balance, why do we need to concern ourselves with this subject at all?

Here's why. The buffering of acids with minerals taken from our tissues is meant to be an occasional backup system, not a constant state of emergency drawdown. When the buffering process becomes an everyday occurrence, we begin to deplete our minerals faster than we replace them. That's what leads to trouble. This phenomenon pops up in this book more than once: our bodies are great at adapting to adverse conditions, but those adaptations sometimes harm us as they help.

We contain more calcium than any other mineral, mostly in our bones and teeth. Sodium and potassium can be found in the interstitial fluids between our cells; magnesium, in our muscles.

Our buffering backup system turns to these minerals when we become too acidic. First, it uses calcium. If we use up a little of that plentiful mineral to buffer acidity, no problem. Especially if we're eating enough of it in our normal diet.

If the buffering becomes a steady drain, though, our calcium content can become depleted. To combat excess acidity, our bodies will produce more calcium, which is just another sign that buffering is required. This is an effective response, but over time it too becomes a source of stress. The result is predictable.

In "Regulation of Bone Cell Function by Acid-Base Balance," *Proceedings of the Nutrition Society, Great Britain*, Jürgen Vormann and Thomas Goedecke reported, "It has been known since the early 20th century that systemic acidosis causes depletion of the skeleton." Vormann and Goedecke also wrote, "In the past, the pH regulation was taken for granted in persons not being severely ill, and the required buffering capacity of the organism was accepted as being virtually inexhaustible. But today latent acidosis resulting from the gradual reduction of the buffer reserves is increasingly in the focus of interest for the development and progression of chronic diseases such as osteoporosis and rheumatoid disorders."

In other words, we are depleting our mineral content to such a degree that we are making ourselves ill with serious diseases.

Excess acidity doesn't just deplete our skeletons, either. One long-term study found that older people who eat an acidic diet will lose more lean muscle mass than those who eat alkaline, plant-based foods. Acidity equals muscle loss. We need all the lean muscle tissue we can get to maintain strength and health as we age.

When we use up sodium and potassium for buffering, we change the environment around our cells for the worse. Those minerals are needed for other important functions, such as regulating the heartbeat, determining the amount of water in our bodies, and developing electrical signals. When we drain magnesium from muscles, we suffer spasms and slower recovery time from injuries. Even as our bodies fight to maintain normal pH, damage is being done. Without sufficient levels of the necessary minerals today, we become vulnerable to chronic, debilitating illnesses in the future.

The symptoms of acidosis—fatigue, lack of energy and motivation, moodiness, headaches, cramps, poor digestion, heartburn, dry skin and hair, and cold hands and feet—are the same minor complaints and everyday aches and pains that people suffer stoically, thinking they can't be helped. Just normal adult life, right?

Wrong. They're not minor problems, and they're not normal. And the fact that lots of other people complain about the same things doesn't mean these conditions are acceptable, let alone inevitable. These are all signs of an overly acidified internal environment, which could mean we're headed for something catastrophic.

But wait—the health food store shelves are filled with calcium supplements. And the supermarket has plenty of food products "fortified" with calcium. We can just replenish the minerals that way, right?

Actually, no. Here's an interesting example of why nutritional supplements aren't always the big fix we wish they were. A recent study measured how well calcium supplements restored the mineral in people with osteoporosis. These people absorbed some of the calcium, the tests showed, but not enough to make a difference. Eating a diet high in mineral-rich vegetables, the study found, got better results in preventing calcium depletion. We can't just eat crap, damage our tissues, and then swallow a pill to make everything better. Pulling a mineral out of its natural state within whole food creates new problems. Instead of rescuing us, that calcium supplement is just one more thing to metabolize.

After researchers from the US Preventive Task Force, part of the Department of Health and Human Services, reviewed existing studies, they published a recommendation against daily supplementation of calcium for the prevention of fractures in postmenopausal women. A study of more than 36,000 postmenopausal women published in the *American Journal of Clinical Nutrition* found that calcium supplementation was associated with an increase in urinary tract stones.

Once again, science proves the wisdom of eating whole foods to get our necessary nutrients. Unlike medication, disease prevention is 100 percent effective, with no harmful side effects.

We can actually use one kind of food to balance out the effects of another. Three servings of an alkalizing food have been found to balance out one serving of something acidifying. That's a rationale for the rule of thumb that says three-quarters of our dinner plates should be covered by vegetables, one-quarter (maximum) by anything else. When we eat an alkaline diet, we are eating the foods that keep every system running as it should.

Without much help from us, our bodies regulate the acid-alkaline balance. But we need to do our part and help maintain a slightly alkaline internal environment, to support the acid buffering system and keep it from draining the minerals we need for everything else.

And everything matters. It's those two coffees as soon as we wake up, giving our bodies a jolt of acidity before we give them anything else. It's the daily highway battle with our fellow commuters, stressing us out and increasing the acidity even further. It's the eight or nine hours nailed to a desk chair, hunched over a computer, and that cheeseburger and sugary soft drink (or even that sugar-free diet version) at lunch, and then a return to highway anxiety and home, with a dinner that features either more animal protein or refined grains in our pasta or pizza, and maybe a drink or two to unwind, followed by a blissful collapse into the sofa. Finish it off with something for that splitting headache and the pills for high cholesterol and blood pressure, then off to bed with an Ambien.

One acidifying event after another. Sure, we ate an apple and a salad and some broccoli, and shot some hoops with the kids. But was that enough to support all the buffering that went on? You know the answer as well as I do.

So we drew down more of our mineral stores without replenishing them. And we forced our kidneys and livers to work a little harder. And we bathed our blood vessels and tissues in a bit more acidity than was good for them.

Now let's multiply this by how many days, weeks, months, years . . .

We alone decide whether we will be acidic and unhealthy, or create the slightly alkaline conditions our bodies need to provide us with a powerful, beautiful vehicle to carry us through our lives.

This is a perfect example of how our culture of medical science fails us. Dr. Warburg discovered the links between acidity and cancer how long ago? More than eighty years. And it's not as though it was a secret—it won him the Nobel Prize! Medical science has known for a long time that no disease, bacteria, or virus can flourish in an alkaline environment, but somehow scientists have failed to make it clear to the rest of us.

Anyway, there's no point crying over the past. What can we do now to help maintain a healthy acid-alkaline balance?

Well, as we've said, our bodies manage that all on their own. But we can use the other four life forces to help.

We've already discussed the crucial role nutrition plays in

restoring minerals. Typically, the people who lose most minerals to the buffering process are the ones who need the best nutrition—and, naturally, the ones not getting it. I suppose we could say that if you insist on eating and drinking poorly, you had better also eat well to make up for it. If you're still having caffeine and alcohol, the yin and yang of artificial stimulation, you should enjoy lots of raw, leafy greens.

In the back of the book, you'll find lists of the most alkalizing and acidifying foods. There's also a list of the foods that contain most minerals. That's a good start. We need to be creative about changing how we eat—we want to have all the things we love best, or why bother eating?

Exercising will bring lots of good oxygen into our bodies, as well as force us to drink plenty of water, both of which help the alkalinity cause. And finally, doing all we can to support our immune systems will at the very least keep our cells clear of any more junk than they already have to deal with.

# Simple To-Do List ✓

- Eat mineral-rich plant foods, and stay away from junk in order to maintain a slightly alkaline internal environment. Our bodies know how to maintain the proper acid-base balance on their own, but we can help by eating healthfully.

- Eat a lot of food raw, every day. Cooking acidifies our food.

- Find ways to eliminate (or at least cut down) the everyday mental strife. Emotional stress also acidifies our tissues by prompting the release of cortisol and other stress responses. Surround yourself with people who inspire you and make you laugh. Speak honestly and truthfully about what is going on in your life.

- Start paying attention not only to food labels but also to the ingredients in your shampoo, body wash, and toothpaste. These industrial chemicals and the preservatives and additives in our food contribute to metabolic acidosis.

# The Protein-Fat Myths

*Too Much of One Good Thing,*
*Not Enough of Another*

P rotein is a wonderful thing.

It performs a lot of important jobs—it builds muscles, organs, and connective tissues, and repairs all those when they need it (which is constantly). Protein is necessary for metabolism and digestion, too. It contributes to the creation of antibodies, which keep us from dying of the infectious germs that surround us at all times. It helps generate energy. Protein is responsible for our protective surfaces, like skin, hair, and nails.

Luckily, protein is easy to come by—it's in practically everything we eat. Meat, fish, and eggs contain quite a bit, of course, and we usually think of them as our main source of this nutrient. But vegetables, beans, grains, nuts, and seeds provide protein, too, just in smaller doses.

Once we consume protein, we break it down into its building blocks, the part we can use—the amino acids. There are twenty-one of these altogether. Our bodies can manufacture a dozen of them, which leaves nine essential amino acids that we need to get totally from outside sources, meaning food.

The human body's need for protein hasn't changed much over the past hundred thousand or so years. But there are trends and fads in nutrition like anything else.

Protein is in style right now.

For a while, we were told that if we wanted to be healthy, we should eat lots of carbs and not so much fat or protein. Eventually somebody noticed that obesity and other metabolic disorders were going through the roof. So the experts reconsidered. No, they said, now cut back on the carbs and eat lots of protein.

Okay, to a point. We need protein, and some people, women and the elderly especially, may not have been getting enough. Increasing protein and cutting carbs will result in better appetite control, for sure. Animal foods that contain it are filling.

But it's a balancing act. Not enough protein, and our bodies don't function properly. Too much, and we run a number of other risks, including excess acidity, which can lead to a long list of dangerous conditions, as we discussed in "Life Force Number Four: Alkalization."

Every day I see recommendations to eat more protein than we need, more than is good for us. It's too much for our bodies to handle. We think we're making ourselves healthy by eating so much protein, but it's having the opposite effect over time. It's making us sicker.

## What Does Excess Protein Harm?

Nitrogen is a wonderful thing too. We need it to help synthesize human proteins, which make up all our tissues plus our DNA, enzymes, hormones, and other important things. Nitrogen is in the air we breathe, but we don't absorb it through our lungs. We ingest it whenever we eat protein. In fact, protein is our only source of nitrogen. (The other components of protein are carbon and hydrogen.)

When we take in too much protein, we end up with more nitrogen than we need. Our bodies don't store it, so we have to excrete it: the pancreas secretes enzymes to break it down, and then the kidneys turn it into urea, and the liver turns it into ammonia. It gets the job done, but these substances are as corrosive to our insides as they sound.

Too much protein also puts us in danger of a buildup of toxic ketones, a condition that puts excess stress on our kidneys as they work to flush them from our bodies. This process uses up so much water that it can cause cellular dehydration, leading to even more difficulties, as we talked about in "Life Force Number Two: Hydration."

"Habitual consumption of excessive dietary protein," according to a study published in the *New England Journal of Medicine*, "negatively impacted kidney function."

When we metabolize protein, it leaves an acidic ash behind. This is how it acidifies our tissues, and it's why our bodies then need buffering with minerals. In 1998 the *Journal of Nutrition* published a study of meat consumption's effect on bone health, which found that "different food proteins differ greatly in their potential acid load, and therefore in their acidogenic [acid-creating] effect. A diet high in acid-ash proteins causes excessive calcium loss." Increasing consumption of fruit and vegetables, the researchers wrote, cuts acid and ammonia production and reduces the loss of calcium in the body. Their conclusion: "Excessive dietary protein from foods with high potential renal acid load adversely affects bone, unless buffered by the consumption of alkali-rich foods or supplements."

Thus protein and the nitrogen it contains, both of which we need, can also harm our health. It's amazing how often this is the case—something that's good for us, even necessary, is bad if we get too much. It's all about the balance.

Mainly, it's the animal-based sources of protein that cause us problems. Vegetables contain protein, too, but you'd have to eat a truckload of kale to get too much protein. When we talk about danger-level hits of protein, we almost always mean meat, poultry, fish, dairy, and eggs. And it's not just the protein that causes problems—it's some of the substances that come along with it.

People rightly point out that we've been eating meat since the earliest days of the species. We thrived and grew strong on it. We love meat. So why worry about it now?

# Too Much Meat

If you pay attention to trends in diet and nutrition, you know that the Atkins program encouraged people to eat as much meat as they wanted. More recently, the Paleo diet said we should eat like the cavemen did, meaning lots of animal protein. The theory is that this is what our Paleolithic ancestors ate; since our bodies haven't evolved much since then, it's what we are built to consume.

People today brag about how much protein they eat, as if it's a medal of honor. Maybe they think that eating lots of flesh makes them seem more powerful and animalistic, like cavemen. The catch is that cavemen had to hunt their meat down, kill it, and drag it home before they could eat it. It wasn't easy. Meat was scarce. At times, *all* food was. That's the environment in which our bodies evolved. We adapted to live under those conditions—not the world as it exists today.

And remember, those ancestors lived only to the ripe old age of thirty or so. They weren't eating for the long haul; they were more worried about making it to tomorrow. And so they ate whatever was available. They couldn't drive to a supermarket loaded with, literally, tons of fresh meat, or pull into a fast-food joint for a quick roadside protein fix. Today meat is so plentiful that we can afford as much as we desire. Back in the Paleolithic era, animal protein was very costly in terms of the energy expenditure required to get some. You had to work for it. You had to burn calories to get calories. If you had a little meat today, you ate it all; there was no guarantee when you'd find some more, and no refrigerator to preserve it for a midnight snack or lunch tomorrow.

When kings are depicted, what are they eating? A big hunk of meat. A huge drumstick. Protein equals power and riches. They're never shown eating a salad, or even a vegetable. Salads are for rabbits, right? In reality, no.

*Scientific American* recently ran an article titled "Human Ancestors Were Nearly All Vegetarians." The author, Rob Dunn, wrote: "Which Paleo diet should we eat? The one from twelve thousand years ago? A hundred thousand years ago? Forty million years ago? If you want to return to your ancestral diet, the one our ancestors ate when most of the features of our guts were evolving, you might reasonably eat what our ancestors spent the most time eating during the largest periods of the evolution of our guts, fruits, nuts, and vegetables—especially fungus-covered, tropical, leaves."

I don't believe we all need to be vegans or even vegetarians to be healthy. But we should be mindful about the animal protein we consume. If we were to limit ourselves to small portions—three to four ounces—of hormone-free, GMO-free organic pasture-raised beef or pork or free-range poultry, maybe this wouldn't be an issue. We could eat it a few times a month—not on a fixed schedule, but only as our bodies need it. But that's not the world of food as it exists today.

Instead of meat scarcity, we've gotten to where some of us get animal protein three times a day—in our breakfast omelet, in our lunchtime sandwich, and then prominently featured on our dinner plates. Does anybody really believe that prehistoric men, women, and kids ate like that?

What are we getting from all that meat and fish? The essential amino acids, for sure. Iron. Some enzymes. B vitamins. Fats. Full bellies.

That's it for the good stuff.

We're also getting a lot of bad stuff—not just increased acidity due to so much protein, but many other harmful substances too.

Meat in the days before agriculture was a whole lot different from what we find today. In those days, animals ate as we humans did—whatever they could forage, all natural and 100 percent wild.

Meat now is plentiful but of lower nutritional quality than ever. It's not even close to what existed before modern ranching and processing. Animals that should be raised on grass are fed grain instead, because it's cheaper. Because of that, we get more omega-6 fats than we should, and not enough omega-3s. When we eat meat today, we are eating the hormones given to the animals to increase yield. We are eating unknown junk used as filler to keep feed costs down. We are eating the antibiotics injected into the animals or included in their food to make them grow bigger and ensure that they stay healthy enough to slaughter. We are eating the fertilizer, pesticides, and herbicides used to grow their feed. We're eating meat from animals kept in horrifying, filthy conditions, virtually guaranteeing that some of us will be stricken with lethal *E. coli* contamination.

Maybe worst of all, we're also eating the genetically modified corn or other grains the animals are fed. Those beasts won't live long enough to suffer any possible side effects from GMOs. But we will. Researchers from the Institute of Health and Environmental Research studied the effects of genetically modified soy and corn in feed on 168 pigs and found that the animals suffered 2.6 times the rate of severe stomach inflammation suffered by pigs given non-GMO feed.

That's meat today—a far cry from what it was even two generations ago. Scientists used to believe it was the saturated animal fat contained in meat that caused most of the health problems. It's a major source of cholesterol, without a doubt. Our blood becomes visibly sludgy when we eat animal fats.

But now we know it's also the bacteria that come along with the fat that causes concern.

A few hours after we eat meat, our blood fills up with endotoxins—poisons—that trigger our immune systems. Something in those animal products causes our bodies to react as though we are under assault from an external invader. Experts now believe that the saturated fat makes our intestinal lining more porous, causing leaky gut syndrome, which we discussed earlier, in "Feeding Our Other Body." It allows digestive bacteria to escape our gut (where it belongs) and enter our bloodstream (where it doesn't).

And those microbes are tough, too. According to a study pub-

lished in 2010 in the *British Journal of Nutrition*, "The ingestion
of fatty meals is associated with a transient, low-grade systemic
inflammatory response in human subjects," and the toxins were
found to be "highly resistant to typical cooking times and temperatures, low pH and protease treatment (enzyme metabolism)."
In other words, they're tough. Cooking doesn't have any effect on
them. Even our digestive juices and enzymes can't neutralize them.

That's why our immune systems respond to animal foods when
they do—not as soon as we've eaten but a few hours later. It's not
just the usual villain, red meat, either—researchers have found
high levels of endotoxins in chicken, pork, dairy, eggs. The endo-
toxin level is lower in wild game, studies have shown, but it still
exists.

The mere fact that our immune systems react to animal-based
food should tell us that it contains something unhealthy for us.
Now, think of how many times most of us have eaten animal foods
over the course of our lives—three times a day, every day, for decades and decades. Remember, this is not only meat, but includes
eggs, cheese, and all dairy. Every meal triggers a new bout of inflammation, which we constantly renew with every plate placed
before us. At some point it becomes a chronic condition. Our
immune systems don't get a breather. Our tissues are always inflamed. This is extremely stressful on the body, which triggers
even more negative conditions. I get into this in "Nutritional
Stress."

This is scary, because researchers today are constantly finding
more connections between inflammation and the signature ailments of our age—cancer, heart disease, obesity, metabolic disorder, osteoporosis, and degenerative diseases like Parkinson's,
multiple sclerosis, and muscular dystrophy. Can we really doubt
that our protein-rich diet is a big part of what's behind these?

And leaky gut is just the beginning.

According to an analysis of research that appeared in
2010 in *Annals of Internal Medicine*, "A low-carbohydrate diet
based on animal sources was associated with higher all-cause

mortality in both men and women, whereas a vegetable-based low-carbohydrate diet was associated with lower all-cause and cardiovascular disease mortality rates."

Meat contains at least three known cancer-causing agents. One is a substance called IGF-1—insulin-like growth factor, a hormone that has been found to cause cancer cells to grow. It's like pouring gasoline on a fire. The other two are heterocyclic amines and nitrosamines, both of which are carcinogens created when animal flesh is cooked. Researchers who looked into how the type of meat and the cooking method influences heterocyclic amine content found that it was highest in fried, well-done meat—3.5 times higher than when meat is eaten medium rare. Bacon had the highest levels, followed by pork, then beef, then chicken.

And a study in the *Journal of Cancer Epidemiology* found that subjects who eat a plant-based diet have a lower circulating level of IGF-1 than meat eaters—13 percent lower in vegans than meat eaters and vegetarians. Leading researcher Naomi Allen stated, "A plant-based diet may be associated with a lower risk of cancer via its effect on IGF-I availability."

The steak house is a favorite feeding place for the red-blooded male of the species. But studies show that when people stop eating meat, their testosterone levels rise. In a recent study for a food-and-cleanse-type program in which subjects gave up meat and dairy for twenty-one days, testosterone levels in men jumped by an average of 30 percent. We may even be losing muscle due to eating meat—researchers have found that a diet rich in vegetables and fruit and low in acidifying protein helps preserve muscle mass in older people.

Meat is the most challenging thing we ask our digestive systems to process. Breaking down muscle fiber of another species into something our bodies can use is hard work—a lot of metabolic stress. If we chew well, we're making meat somewhat easier to process. Still, it hangs around in our stomachs longer than any other food. If we mix meat with other things—vegetables, say, or bread or grains—the situation gets even worse. Now our digestive efforts are being diverted away from the meat, meaning it will lie around in there even longer, putrefying. (Meaning that if we do eat meat, we should finish it first, before the other foods.)

Eating meat has been associated with increased risk of Crohn's disease, irritable bowel syndrome, and even urinary tract infections. The latest research shows we can get the bacteria from poultry without even eating it: one study showed that just being in the same room as chicken while it's being prepared or eaten can contaminate us with the harmful germs it contains. Scary, right? Meat also harbors parasites, which are involved in many of the diseases we suffer.

And the problem isn't just that we're eating the meat from unhealthy animals. The abuse of antibiotics is creating strains of drug-resistant germs that can sicken animals and humans alike, according to a report from the Pew Commission on Industrial Farm Animal Production, a joint project of the Pew Charitable Trusts and the Johns Hopkins Bloomberg School of Public Health. An analysis of that study performed by the Johns Hopkins Center for a Livable Future stated, "Many of the drugs used in this context are no different from those used in human medicine. In the context of food animal production, the use of antimicrobials continues to increase steadily and greatly surpasses uses in humans. Administering non-therapeutic antimicrobials to food animals is particularly problematic since chronic administration of low doses of antimicrobials contributes to the evolution and proliferation of antimicrobial-resistant strains of bacteria."

Sound appetizing? That's what we eat when we eat meat. Skinless chicken breasts, even. True, it's possible to buy "clean" meat, meaning from animals raised on organic grass, free ranging and without hormones, antibiotics, or adulterated feed. But it's so expensive and hard to find that it's out of reach for most of us. That's not such a bad thing—it would ensure that we don't overdo it. The only other alternative: raise it, kill it, and butcher it yourself.

Finally, meat is contributing to our national weight problem. An eight-year study published in the *Journal of the American Society for Nutrition* surveyed more than 300,000 people in ten European countries and found that an intake of 250 grams of conventionally raised meat led to a weight increase of nearly a pound a year. The lead researcher wrote, "Our results indicate that meat intake is positively associated with weight gain during adult life in [European] subjects."

Even from the anthropological point of view, our status as meat eaters is in doubt. William C. Roberts, editor in chief of the *American Journal of Cardiology* and medical director of the Baylor University Heart and Vascular Institute, in the red-blooded state of Texas, says that humans aren't physiologically designed to be meat eaters. Our intestinal length, our need for vitamin C from outside sources, and our ability to sweat link us more closely to herbivorous than to carnivorous mammals. "I think the evidence is pretty clear," he says. "If you look at various characteristics of carnivores versus herbivores, it doesn't take a genius to see where humans line up."

Our flat (rather than pointed) teeth, the carb-metabolizing enzyme amylase contained in our saliva, and the fact that we, unlike carnivores, can't metabolize uric acid also suggest that we are better adapted to eat plants than animal foods. The health benefits of plants, and the evidence that animal foods can harm us, only make the choices clearer.

It may take science years or even decades to prove, once and for all, all the ways that eating animal foods hurts us over time. I would rather not wait to find out before I take the hint. I stopped eating meat because not eating it makes me feel better, but I had to try living without it before I knew for sure. And that's really the bottom line: we each need to try different foods, and new ways of thinking about what we eat. How else can we discover what works best for us, individually?

# How Much Protein Is Safe?

So what can we do to avoid all that potential damage?

The obvious answer is to lighten up on the protein—to get all we need, but no more. Unfortunately, there's no consistent advice out there on how much protein is healthy for us. Even reputable sources of nutritional information tell us to eat too much. It's going to come back to haunt us.

Some so-called experts recommend that we get between 25 and 30 percent of our daily calories from protein. For most of us, that's too much to eat on a regular basis. Your needs may rise or fall, depending on your activity levels or what else you're eating. Many people are unaware of this interesting fact: our bodies actually recycle and reuse somewhere between 100 and 300 grams of protein daily—yet more evidence that we evolved in a world where protein was scarce. According to scientists, we excrete only around 6 percent of the protein we ingest every day. The rest remains with us. We have more protein available than we realize.

I believe we should be eating around one-third of a gram of protein for every pound of body weight. A 150-pound person should get around 50 grams a day, or a little under two ounces.

What contains two ounces of protein? Top round beef is about one-third protein, so a six-ounce steak equals *all* the protein our 150-pound person needs in a day. An egg contains 12.5 grams of protein, so four eggs would be enough, even if you didn't get another bit from anything else you ate. Two four-ounce skinless chicken breasts provide just under 50 grams. Same for two cans of tuna.

Or we could get most or all of our protein from nonflesh sources—vegetables, legumes, whole grains, nuts, seeds, and some dairy, like yogurt.

Let's imagine a day where, among other things, we eat

almonds, hummus, spinach, brown rice, kale, yogurt, peas, black beans, and pumpkin seeds. One ounce of almonds equals roughly 6 grams of protein. Three ounces of hummus contains 7.4 grams. Three ounces of spinach contains 2.8 grams. In one cup of kale, 2 grams. In a cup of black beans, 14.5 grams. In a cup of brown rice, 5 grams. Peas, 7.5 grams per cup. Pumpkin seeds, 6 grams per half cup. And let's throw in a little nutrient-dense quinoa, worth about 8 grams of protein per cooked cup.

There—all the protein we need in a day, about 50 grams, from nutrient-dense, whole healthy foods. Foods that give us many other beneficial things as well, and little metabolic stress. We could come up with an entirely different list of foods and end up with the same amount of healthy protein, and without any of the saturated fats or other sketchy substances found in meat, fish, and eggs.

Here's another way to compute it: somewhere between 10 and 15 percent of our total calories should come from protein. If we're eating 2,000 calories a day, that's around 200 or 300 calories' worth of protein.

There are any number of formulas I can pass along that will allow us to measure precisely how much protein we should be eating a day. But let me ask you something: Do you really want to go to all that trouble? You need to be a mathematician-nutritionist to compute the exact amount of protein you need to eat to stay healthy. You'd have to weigh everything you're about to consume, and then look up its nutritional values, to plan a meal.

Who wants to go through life that way? Luckily, we don't have to, as long as we get most if not all our protein from plant sources.

Plant protein is accompanied by vitamins, minerals, enzymes, phytonutrients, and other beneficial chemicals. So even though the protein acidifies us, all the rest of that stuff alkalizes our bodies. We're getting amino acids with no cost to the acid-alkaline balance. Look at kale, for instance—51 percent protein, almost as much as a steak per weight, and yet its overall influence is alkalizing because of the calcium and other minerals it contains.

Of course, meat is a whole lot denser than kale. One hundred calories of steak is about one ounce, compared to twelve ounces of kale. So you need big portions of food when you're getting protein from vegetable sources. This should be good news for people who fear that they'll starve if they have to live on a healthy diet. Once you cut out the harmful foods, you really have to eat a lot.

But wait, you say—kale is not a *complete* protein. Meaning, it does not contain all nine essential amino acids we require. That's a common misconception. In fact, kale *does* contain all nine essential amino acids, just not as much as meat has.

But it's true that some vegetables do not have all nine amino acids that we need to get from food sources. However, if our diet includes a wide variety of plant foods—as many different kinds of vegetable, nut, seed, and bean as we can manage—then we will get all the essential amino acids. Having the same four vegetables over and over, prepared in the same exact way, won't cut it. Neither will having just a side dish of zucchini or the occasional lettuce and tomato salad. You've got to really commit to your vegetables. Even romaine lettuce has protein!

Also, plant-based foods contain lots of water, which we need for digestion and many other purposes. Meat is dense and consumes water rather than contributing it.

How about our immune systems—how do they respond to plant-based foods? As a matter of fact, vegetables and fruit contain substances that are toxic to the creatures (humans included) who eat them. We discussed this earlier—plants develop toxins, irritants, and other phytochemicals to keep their predators from overfeeding. It's a survival mechanism. Everything that lives wishes to survive. Some of these, in excess, can actually cause us digestive distress. That's the reason we want to eat a wide variety of foods—to keep from getting too much of any individual toxin.

Still, our cells recognize vegetables as being nutritious, beneficial, and bio-available. That's how our bodies express their preference.

We can guarantee we're getting enough protein and all the other nutrients if we just eat a varied diet of vegetables, legumes, nuts, and seeds. Today, when excess weight has become our number-one health obsession, this is a plan that requires us to eat a *lot* of food every day. In fact, if we eat too little, we put our health at risk. And it's virtually impossible to eat too much.

I think we all ought to consider cutting back on meat, if not giving it up altogether. For a lot of people this is going to sound impossible. Until not so long ago, I ate meat every day. And I was extremely healthy. Today I work out harder than I ever have in my life, and I'm even healthier than before, without any animal protein in my diet.

I'm a muscular guy, and I lift weights and work my body pretty hard, so I get this question all the time: "How can you get enough protein if you don't eat meat, or fish?" It's easy. Have some beans, nuts, spinach, kale or quinoa, and you'll get all you need. Throw some chickpeas, quinoa, or pumpkin seeds in with your salad, and you will get a big load of other healthy nutrients too, with none of the nutritional or metabolic stress that comes from eating meat. If I feel the need for more protein, I don't go out looking for that alone. I just eat more of everything. That will provide all the protein I need. And I don't have to stress over it. Eat healthy food, and our bodies will do the rest.

A steak is 32 percent protein. Spinach is 31 percent. The steak is calorie-dense. The spinach is nutrient-dense. Which sounds like the better choice?

Here, I've listed the protein contained in some common foods. (For each, I'm giving grams of protein per 100 grams of food, roughly 3.5 ounces.)

HARD-BOILED EGG: 12.5 grams

ROASTED ALMONDS: 21 grams

A BIG MAC: 12 grams

ROASTED HAZELNUTS: 15 grams

BROILED T-BONE STEAK: 24–27 grams, depending on the leanness

PEANUT BUTTER: 25 grams

SKINLESS CHICKEN BREAST: 33 grams

ROASTED PUMPKIN SEEDS: 18.5 grams

BROWN RICE: 2.5 grams

COOKED QUINOA: 4.4 grams (raw quinoa is 14 grams!)

AVOCADO: 2 grams

SWEET POTATO, BAKED IN SKIN: 2 grams

BLACK BEANS: almost 9 grams

HUMMUS: 8 grams

RAW SPINACH: 2.8 grams

LENTILS: 9 grams

TOFU: 9 grams

You get the idea. It's possible to get all the protein and essential amino acids we need from plant-based foods. I hope by now I've shown that it's not as hard as some people make it seem.

Over the years I've heard many people say, "Oh, I tried going vegetarian, but it just didn't work for me." I always want to ask, "Gee, how hard did you try?" Just giving up meat doesn't make you a vegetarian; it just makes you a poorly nourished person—unless you actually do all the other things necessary to be a healthy non-meat eater. It's entirely possible to eat a vegetarian diet that is unhealthy, unnutritious, and generally lousy. People do it all the time, and then decide that living without meat just doesn't work for them. It's crazy. You could live on Oreos, potato chips, pasta, and grape soda and still call yourself a vegan. Our bodies are our best feedback mechanisms.

We can't just give up meat and fish and expect to magically, automatically become properly fed. We need to work at it a little. We need to shop differently. Preparing our food takes more time, effort, and thought. We have to pay attention to what we're eating, make sure we're getting all the right nutrients. This is especially true when it comes to protein. We make sure to get a variety of greens, beans, seeds. We can no longer just throw a big steak into the frying pan, or sauté a chicken breast, and add a potato and a little broccoli on the side and call that a meal. The traditional idea of what constitutes dinner goes out the window. We have to take responsibility for what goes into our mouths. No more autopilot. Take time to form new habits, and then it will be no big deal—and you will feel better because of it.

It's work. But all good things are.

Just as one food fad has led us to consume more protein than we should, another has caused us to fear fat as if it were a harmful substance. But it's not.

Most foods—even plants—contain fats. Fat is one of our three basic nutrients, along with protein and carbs. It makes up a critical part of every one of our cells. It provides us with essential fatty acids, which are not present in the body and must be gotten from food. These are important for controlling inflammation, blood clotting, and brain development. Our brains are 60 percent fat! Our bodies can't absorb certain vitamins unless fat is present. It's also a source of energy.

If we don't eat fats, we don't live. Can't get any more important than that.

Maybe it's just that we confuse nutritional fat with body fat. For a while, the supermarket shelves were filled with foods—mostly unhealthy ones, like cookies and other processed items—boasting that they were "low-fat" or "fat free." We took that to mean they were good for us, and would help us control our weight. Just the opposite was true, since when they took out the fat, they added sugars and other junk. We began consuming epic amounts of refined carbs—bread, pasta, and anything else made from wheat. As a result, we ended up with insulin resistance, high triglycerides, and even more body fat. The unhealthy standard American diet exists partly because of our irrational fear of fat.

We were also told to avoid certain fats because they would cause cardiovascular disease by blocking our arteries with cholesterol. Today, our understanding of fat and heart health is changing rapidly. Scientists are finding more and more evidence that fat isn't as dangerous as was previously believed. In fact, they're now reminding us that it's a necessary part of a healthy diet.

Finally, there's the fact that, ounce for ounce, fats have more calories than either protein or carbs. That probably scared people off most of all. It's easy to see how we've gotten so mixed up. No wonder fats became practically taboo.

The first thing we need to remember is that there *are* bad fats—ones that harm our health and provide no benefits. By now, most of us are aware that trans fats and hydrogenated fats are highly processed, completely man-made and unnatural, and impossible for our bodies to metabolize without damage. These have been linked to heart disease and diabetes, and should be shunned as though they are poison. You find them among the long lists of ingredients in processed foods, and they're often used to cook fast food and other cheap grub. Lots of products and restaurant chains now boast that they no longer use these fats, and I suspect they'll disappear before long.

But it's not as simple as bad fats or good ones.

For example, all fats occurring naturally in foods are either saturated or unsaturated. The terms are meaningful only to chemists—it has to do with whether the carbon molecules in fat are saturated with hydrogen or not. Doesn't matter for our purposes. We need both kinds.

Saturated fat typically comes from animal sources—meat, butter, milk, cheese—though coconut oil and palm oil contain it too. We need saturated fats for our cell membranes, our immune systems, and other important functions. But these have also been tagged with a big red warning label. Scientists pointed out that saturated fats contain LDLs—low-density lipoproteins—which are also known as "bad" cholesterol, the kind that clogs up our arteries and leads to heart attack.

For that reason, these were thought of as "bad" fats, too. For years, the heart experts told us we should get a tiny amount, no more than 5 percent of our daily calories, of saturated fats—the equivalent of two tablespoons of butter.

But recent research has begun questioning that anti-saturated-fat gospel. In 2014 a huge analysis of data involving seventy-six studies and half a million subjects was published in *Annals of Internal Medicine*. It found that people who ate higher amounts of saturated fat had no more heart disease than those who ate less. And it didn't find less heart disease in people who ate the supposedly healthier unsaturated fats from plant sources, such as olive oil.

As you can imagine, this jolted scientists and cardiologists, challenging what had been rock-solid beliefs about fat and heart health. If saturated fat wasn't creating all that bad cholesterol, what was? It now appears that sugar and refined carbs may be the main culprits. Quite a turnaround.

So now what? I believe we should get 10 to 15 percent of our daily calories from saturated fats. If we're obtaining it from animal sources, we need to take care that they are clean, meaning not accompanied by the harmful substances we discussed earlier in this chapter. Meat ought to be grass-fed and raised with no pesticides and no antibiotics or hormones. It should not come from meat factories—the animals should be raised and slaughtered humanely, which makes their meat safer for us, too. If we're not eating meat, we can get saturated fat from whole-food sources like raw pastured organic butter and organic coconut oil.

Traditionally, the experts have tried to steer us toward unsaturated fats from plant sources. These were the healthy ones, we were told, the fats that created high-density lipoproteins—the good cholesterol. These fats are classified as either monounsaturated or polyunsaturated, another distinction that doesn't really matter as far as we're concerned. The main thing is that we get these fats fresh, because once they turn rancid, they create more harmful free radicals we have to deal with. These fats should be clean, well tested, properly packaged, and stored for our safety.

Good sources of monounsaturated fats include nuts, oils from nuts (such as almonds, macadamias, cashews), olive oil, avocados, flaxseed, and sesame seeds or oil, to name a few. We can get enough of these fats as long as we eat a healthy diet.

The polyunsaturated fats include our sources of essential fatty acids, EFAs—*essential* meaning that we need them, but our bodies don't have them, so we *must* eat foods that enable us to synthesize them.

And this leads us to yet another distinction: omega-3 and omega-6 EFAs. We need both; that's why they're called essential. They are among the most biologically active nutrients in our bodies. The main thing to remember is that we need to get them in the proper ratio.

Most of us already get plenty of omega-6 EFAs, from foods such as grains, vegetable oils, poultry, and eggs. It's found in lots of processed foods, especially those using soybean oil and palm oil. The meat of animals fed on grains instead of grass contains lots of omega-6 fats, yet another reason to eat meat in moderation, if at all.

Meanwhile, most of us don't consume enough omega-3s, which are found in fish, walnuts, algae, flaxseed, chia seeds, and green plants. The proper intake ratio should be around two parts omega-6 to one part omega-3. There's evidence that prehistoric people thrived on a ratio of 1:1. But most people today get somewhere between 10:1 and 25:1.

The most important omega-3 fatty acids are known by their initials—EPA and DHA (the full chemical names are about half a mile long). Both are critical to brain function especially, but also benefit heart health and joints. Even though we can get these from cold-water fish like mackerel, herring, and anchovies, we probably won't get enough. Thus we almost certainly need to supplement.

Fish oil capsules are practical because the fish have already converted the fats into a form our bodies can use. The problem with fish oil, of course, is the same as the problem with fish: they have been so tainted by mercury, heavy metals, PCBs, radioactivity, and other toxins, thanks to how we've polluted the rivers and seas, that they have to be consumed cautiously, if at all. That's why omega-3s from plant sources are probably the way to go.

Beyond that, we should just stick with the same wisdom we've been discussing all along: Eat whole foods, a wide variety of them, and make sure they're fresh and clean and from trustworthy sources. Do that, and we'll get what we need.

# Simple To-Do List ✓

- Get no more than about 15 percent of a day's total calories from protein. We can get all the protein we need—and the essential amino acids—from plant sources. It's healthier for a number of reasons, chiefly because animal protein today comes with a lot of unhealthy baggage. Those vegetables and beans include many healthy nutrients and antioxidants along with the protein they contain.

- If you want protein from animal foods, organic free-range eggs are the healthiest source. If you eat meat, it should be in small portions of pasture-raised, non-GMO, organic grass-fed (in the case of beef, pork, and lamb), and without the hormones and antibiotics used on factory farms. Eat only fish that is wild-caught, and in modest portions.

- Eat salads that contain a great source of plant-based fat, some nuts or seeds, or at least a dressing made with a little oil. Without fat present, we can't absorb certain nutrients. Even butter, scientists now agree, can be a healthy source of fat, as long as it is from organically fed, pastured cows.

- Steer clear of trans fats and anything labeled "partially hydrogenated," which will someday be banned from all food, I believe.

- Cut back on the omega-6 essential fatty acids, which are commonly found in animal foods, processed foods, junk food, and in palm and canola oils, and increase the amount of healthy omega-3 fats in your diet.

# Nutritional Stress

Back in "Life Force Number One: Nutrition," we talked about the importance of feeding our cells the things they need. But we have to be just as careful about what they *don't* need. Because feeding our cells what they don't need can harm them—meaning us—by impairing their normal functioning.

In other words, cells get stressed like anybody else.

What don't our cells need? We know they require water, electrolytes, oxygen, fats, amino acids, and all those nutrients that keep us alive and well. Anything that doesn't fit that category is by definition unnecessary as far as our cells are concerned. They perceive it as a foreign intruder, and therefore as a threat.

I'm talking about food that harms us, engineered and processed in ways that make it the opposite of nutritious—antinutrients, you could say. That's really an example of the world turned upside down. Crazy!

But today it's the most commonplace thing around. Go to the supermarket or the fast-food restaurant or the soda vending machine. Many of the ingredients started out as nutritious—fruit, water, nuts, vegetables—but were processed and transformed into something quite different. It's edible, so it qualifies as food, but it's not food in any other meaningful way. It doesn't sustain us, support our bodies, fuel our functions, or endow our health. Instead, it's laden with harmful substances—preservatives, additives, chemical dyes and flavorings.

We still call it food, but by now that's a label, not a description.

Not that this stops all of us from eating it. We talk about eating disorders, meaning anorexia and bulimia, which affect just a tiny percentage of people. But all around us are those with the unmistakable symptom of a serious eating disorder—they're unhealthy.

One definition of *eating disorder* is the knowing consumption of things that will hurt us and cut short our lives. It's the kind of behavior we see every day. Every TV commercial for a big chain restaurant routinely promotes "food" that we all know is damaging rather than life-giving fuel. We don't even notice, it's become such a part of everyday life. *That*'s an eating disorder. We pay companies to take perfectly good water and then adulterate it with refined sugar and other harmful sweeteners, dye, chemical flavoring agents, and acidifying artificial carbonation. Then we buy it and drink it—*that's* an eating disorder.

Blame our bad food culture for how normal it all seems. Once upon a time, there was a single food culture. We all carried around a pretty similar idea of what constituted a good meal, how food should be prepared, and where and with whom it was eaten. Today we have two food cultures: good and bad.

Last time I watched TV, I saw a commercial for a restaurant serving pancakes topped with whipped cream topped with canned fruit topped with syrup. It was immediately followed by a commercial for a chain of cancer treatment centers. The bad food culture has become such a part of our lives that we don't even notice how the first commercial's product is creating the demand for the second commercial's service. It's so perfectly self-contained, it's insane.

Meanwhile, we keep on consuming things that we know cause disease and early death. We even feed them to our kids. That's *really* an eating disorder.

# What Causes Nutritional Stress?

According to Brendan Brazier's excellent book *Thrive*, nutritional stress is "created by food because of its unhealthy properties."

Let's start with the obvious stuff.

Refined sugar. Doesn't get any more obvious than that.

Sugar is a poison, absolutely toxic to the body. The definition of poison is, according to *Merriam-Webster*, "a substance that through its chemical action usually kills, injures, or impairs an organism." Hello, sugar.

We need sugar, true, but we can easily get all we require from fruit, vegetables, dairy. That's plenty to satisfy our requirement for glucose as a source of energy. The bad stuff is what nutritionists call "added sugar"—meaning refined sugar and its evil cousin, high-fructose corn syrup. Completely, 100 percent unnecessary as far as our cells are concerned.

Dr. Robert Lustig is a specialist in pediatric hormone disorders and an expert on childhood obesity who teaches at the University of California–San Francisco School of Medicine. He has probably done more than anyone to sound the alarm on sugar. "Added sweeteners," he wrote, "pose dangers to health that justify controlling them like alcohol." And sugar's damage isn't just because it makes us fat, he says. "It has nothing to do with the calories. It's a poison by itself."

Consuming sugar has been linked to cancer, heart disease, high blood pressure, stroke, diabetes, metabolic syndrome, depression, and of course obesity. It taxes our livers, which must process it (they turn it into body fat). Too much of that, and our livers become fatty, too, impairing their ability to do all their other important jobs, like detoxification. Sugar acidifies our tissues, which, as we saw in "Life Force Number Four: Alkalization," is itself a cause of disease. Just as sugar creates harmful spikes in insulin production, dangerously overtaxing the pancreas, it also prompts increased output of serotonin, the feel-good brain chemical. This partly explains why we love sugar so much—eating it makes us high. Too much of that, and we crash, causing brain fatigue, which drives us to desire more sugar.

The harm done by high-fructose corn syrup, which is found in everything from candy bars to sliced bread, doesn't stop with how it causes obesity. Duke University Medical Center studied a group of more than four hundred adults and found that nearly 80 percent of them suffered abnormal liver activity when consuming products containing high-fructose corn syrup. "We found that increased consumption of high-fructose corn syrup was associated with scarring in the liver, or fibrosis, among patients with non-alcoholic fatty liver disease," said the study's lead researcher. Considering that an estimated 30 percent of the U.S. population suffers from nonalcoholic fatty liver disease, this is a serious public health concern.

Bodywide, sugar causes volatility in all our systems, which just adds to the stress, prompting the release of the hormone cortisol. That's helpful in small doses but harmful in prolonged exposure, like when we are chronically stressed—which is precisely what happens when we make sugar a daily part of our diet. Chronic stress equals chronic inflammation, which is the same thing as being sick 100 percent of the time. That's sugar.

Too much cortisol causes hypertension and suppresses thyroid function. It acidifies our tissues and increases the storage of abdominal fat while decreasing our immunity. A deadly cycle can develop: an impaired immune system leads to increased risk of disease; disease damages nutritional status; compromised nutritional status further impairs immunity. Chronically high cortisol can cause cravings for sugar, salt, and fat. When we satisfy those hungers, we worsen nutrient stress, and yet another harmful cycle begins.

Sugar, or sucrose, starts out as a plant—sugarcane is just a variety of tall grass—but it has been stripped of its fiber, protein, vitamins, minerals, lipids, and antioxidants. It was once part of a complex structure, but then it was isolated, crystallized, changed into pure sweetness. Pure poison.

Additionally, the more calories we get from sugar, the less we're likely to get from healthy foods. So the damage is doubled.

The worst part is how difficult it is nowadays to escape sugar. Food manufacturers find a way to put it in everything, even where it has no business. These corporations know how to profit from our addiction. This is a big reason every expert on health tells us to avoid processed foods.

Okay, so let's say we get the message that sugar is bad for us. What do we do about it? Find a way to live without everything being so sweet? Not always, unfortunately. Often we just replace the sugar with sweetening chemicals. Take diet soda, for instance. People drink it thinking they've made a healthier choice. But they're wrong. For one thing, diet drinks encourage us to keep seeking out sweet tastes, which inevitably leads us back to sugar. In fact, a study found that when our bodies get that sweet taste but zero calories to accompany it, they feel cheated. It drives us to drink more, hoping for the high-caloric payoff of real sugar.

And when you drink something containing an artificial sweetener, you're taking in a toxic substance. The most popular one, aspartame, is actually mind-altering, research has shown—it's what scientists call an "excitotoxin." Aspartame has been found, in lab tests on mice, to create brain lesions. Doesn't sound like such a healthy choice, does it? Our cells don't recognize it as a food or anything they can use, so it is treated as a hostile invader, something that must be filtered, neutralized, and excreted. More work for our kidneys and liver. If they're already overworked, the toxin may end up stored in our adipose fat. When those fat cells die, the toxins will still be hanging around.

Imagine now this scenario happening over and over again, many times a day, week after month after year, as we ingest dyes, flavorings, preservatives, and all the other nonfood ingredients found in anything packaged or processed—phony stuff that makes our bodies a little phonier. Then add pesticides, herbicides, fungicides, and larvicides from conventionally grown produce, hormones and antibiotics from conventionally raised livestock, and the petrochemicals and other harmful substances that leach into our food from plastic and metal containers. Every day we add a bit more poison to our systems. We're feeding ourselves things that are actually damaging our nutritional profile, doing the exact opposite of what nutrition is supposed to do. They're even undoing the benefits of our healthy eating.

*That's* nutritional stress.

If instead of that soft drink we crack open a coconut and drink the water in it, our bodies recognize every drop of it—all the nutrients, all the incredible good things in it—and take it in, using it to benefit us. Plus, it tastes great.

Of course we can't find a coconut in every vending machine we come across in the course of a day. There's not a cooler full of them in the convenience store. And getting a drink from a coconut involves a bit more work than opening a can of diet whatever.

Better, then, to stick with water, and steer clear of sugar.

# Bread Is a Sugar-Delivery System

Here's another obvious source of major nutrient stress, nearly as bad as sugar: processed grains. These are grains, wheat mostly, that have been stripped of their fiber and, with it, whatever nourishment they once contained. Which wasn't all that much to begin with—even whole grains don't contain a lot of the nutrients our bodies require. Nothing we can't get in abundance from other plant-based sources.

Even in their natural state, some whole grains contain self-protective substances like phytic acid or enzyme inhibitors that may cause digestive problems in any creature that eats them, including us. These antinutrients can be neutralized if we treat the grains first—soak them, sprout them, or ferment them. Some food makers have begun taking these steps to make whole grains safer for us to eat.

Once the grain has been refined, however, it turns into something just a step away from sugar. Our bodies convert it into glucose pretty quickly, which is why anything made with wheat flour carries such a big glycemic load. It causes the same spike in insulin as sugar does, meaning that it also contributes to insulin resistance, acidosis, pancreatic fatigue, and metabolic syndrome. The proteins in the gluten can lead to leaky gut syndrome, celiac disease, and other major causes of digestive system stress.

The one thing grains have going for them is that they are cheap to produce. If it's a choice between eating food made with refined, processed flour and starving to death, by all means have the flour. Otherwise, best to stay away.

Could bread, pasta, pizza, crackers, and cereal really be so bad for us? Dr. David Ludwig, director of the New Balance Foundation Obesity Prevention Center at Children's Hospital Boston, says, "Refined carbohydrates, including refined grain products, are the single most harmful influence in the American diet today." That sounds pretty bad to me.

Still, we love to eat everything possible on a white bun or sliced bread. It's convenient as hell. The entire fast-food kingdom is built on bread. But eating it means that we are constantly getting hits of sugar mixed in with the unhealthy fats and the excessive protein. Look at the list of ingredients in your typical loaf of bread. You will almost surely find sugar, high-fructose corn syrup, and maybe even plain old corn syrup, too—three kinds of sugar, in addition to the worthless refined wheat flour.

It's not bread, it's a sugar-delivery system. Same is true for pasta.

Refined sugar and refined grains are major sources of nutrient stress—a huge chunk of what's wrong with the standard American diet. If they alone were eliminated from what we eat, our health would make a dramatic, instant improvement.

## The Rest of the Sources

By now most of us have read about the supposed links between high salt intake and hypertension. But keep in mind that the re-fined salt found in processed foods isn't the same thing as the necessary sodium we get from sources like unrefined crystal salt, which contains electrolytes, like Himalayan crystal salt. We need salt to live—and, contrary to what we've all been told, salt in itself doesn't cause high blood pressure. But when we get too much salt and not enough water or potassium, hypertension may be the result.

The solution isn't to eliminate salt. We just need to consume unrefined crystal salt only, along with sufficient potassium (from whole foods) and water. Remember, salt is food. It can be of good quality or bad. Eat natural sources, as unprocessed as we can find. Once again, if we rely on whole foods and water, we will remain healthy and balanced.

Excess protein causes nutritional stress. We've discussed that elsewhere in this book—more than once, I know—but it bears repeating. Any more than 15 percent of our daily calories in protein is more than we need. The protein itself is a problem, and if it comes from animal sources, it is accompanied by even more sources of nutritional stress—harmful bacteria, hormones, chemicals. Whatever junk they fed those poor beasts is now a part of your meal, too. You just can't see it.

Another invisible source of nutrient stress: genetically modified organisms. The Europeans are way ahead of us on recognizing the threats that come from seeds and plants that have been altered at the DNA level in the lab. According to an article published by scientists at the University of Athens Medical School, "The results of most studies with GM [genetically modified] foods indicate that they may cause some common toxic effects such as hepatic, pancreatic, renal, or reproductive effects and may alter the hematological, biochemical, and immunologic parameters."

Today, GMOs are a red-hot battleground. Food activists are working to force the corporations to label products made using genetically modified organisms. The companies, for obvious reasons, are fighting any regulation that would require them to tell us what we're eating.

Are you a smoker or a toker? Are you taking prescription drugs? Drinking coffee in the morning and wine at night? All those contribute to the stress caused by things we consume. The more chemicals we take in, the more good nutrition we need just to counter all the badness. You already know all this. I'm just giving you a nudge and asking you to be a little more honest about it.

Consider this: research conducted by the federal Centers for Disease Control says that 53 percent of the people who die prior to age sixty-five do so "for reasons directly related to lifestyle."

I guess a bowl of potato chips from time to time or a good bottle of wine and maybe a steak with friends are okay. We definitely benefit from fun and happy times. But if we do it every day, or even every week? Not so good.

# The Results of Nutritional Stress

Something new enters our bloodstream, making its way to all our cells, and our bodies have to figure it out and respond to it. If there are chemicals they don't recognize, our bodies immediately begin to react. Antibodies and antigens are triggered. Oxidation of cells occurs. Eat real, 100 percent food, and what happens? The body looks at that raw baby kale and says, "This I recognize! I know what to do with it." There's nothing to buffer or neutralize, and overall, less energy is used to digest and metabolize, meaning less stress.

Of course nobody can survive solely on raw baby kale salad. But the more foods like that we eat, the less stress we create inside our bodies. It is exponentially healthier to eat fruit than Froot Loops.

Today, we produce many more reactive molecules than ever before. But oxidative reactions and the creation of life-saving antioxidants happen as a natural part of metabolizing what we eat. We keep those two forces in balance by eating whole, natural foods. If we eat lousy food instead, we haven't gotten the antioxidants we need. And as a result of all that poor nutrition, we need them more than ever. Instead, we're using up the ones we have, thereby unleashing a tsunami of free radicals.

Anytime we eat nonfood, our bodies are stressed. But we are strong and can adapt to almost anything—for a while. In a way, we'd be better off if that weren't true. If our insides rebelled at once, we'd have to start eating better. But our bodies are loyal soldiers. They will take whatever abuse we throw at them and keep marching as though nothing were wrong.

Then we wake up one day and say, Oh no, why do I have heart disease, or cancer? The answer is obvious, whether or not we wish to see it. Was it our genetics? No, probably not. It was all those years we spent eating and drinking junk. Maybe we thought we were getting away with it, but we weren't; it just took a while. It operated on body time, which we can't fathom.

We need to make a habit of asking: Is this food clean? Does it contain pesticides, herbicides, other industrial chemicals? Was it made with GMOs? Was it created in a kitchen or a factory? Are the few recognizable ingredients accompanied by a long list of additives, flavorings, preservatives, colorings, weird-sounding chemicals, none of which we would ever voluntarily eat? Our bodies need to digest and metabolize every one of them, not just the nutrients.

The list of things that can trigger nutritional stress is nearly endless. The majority of stresses we endure aren't emotional or psychological ones; they come from unhealthy food and drink— bad habits. The main principle to keep in mind is this: anything our bodies don't recognize as food will be a source of stress on our systems. When it comes to eating, every choice counts. Want to lower the stress levels in your life, and add many positive side effects to boot? Eat mostly whole plant foods!

There are people who think that a fast-food dollar-menu meal is a better value than a salad of organic fruit and vegetables. But there may come a day when that dollar meal will be the costliest thing you ever ate.

# Simple To-Do List

- Cut out the two most common, most harmful sources of nutritional stress: added sugar and refined grains. Do this, and you're instantly taking a big step toward eliminating the harm that comes from things you eat.

- Don't replace sugar with artificial sweetener. These chemicals confuse our metabolism and cause us to store fat improperly, and are toxic to our brains and other organs. Use natural concentrated sweeteners such as stevia, luo han gao, coconut flower sugar, or dates.

- Avoid eating anything that cells don't need for healthy functioning. Most often, this means processed foods, which contain substances not found in nature and not really needed by the human body. Stick with whole, plant-based foods.

- Eat unrefined salt. Himalayan crystal salt costs a little more than the supermarket kind, and is a little harder to find, but is worth seeking out. Refined salt is another source of nutritional stress. This is the kind found in snack foods and other junk. Remember, unrefined salt is full of needed electrolytes. It's cellular food!

- Avoid pesticides, herbicides, and GMOs used to grow our fruits and vegetables. Even when we try to eat healthy, we can be dosed with bad stuff. If we grow our own food or get it from trusted farmers' markets and cook it at home, we take total control of what goes into our bodies.

# Life Force Number Five: Detoxification

We've all seen news video from cities where the trash collectors go on strike.

At first the plastic bags line the curbs. Then they pile up into small mountains and spill over, forcing pedestrians to walk in the gutter. The bags rip, and the contents pour out, clogging the sidewalks and making everything disgusting. Then bugs and other vermin begin to feast, spreading filth and disease. The mountains grow taller and broader until no one can get around them—not that you'd want to try. By this point the aroma is pretty funky, and there's a lot of weird stuff in the air. Everything is buried beneath the garbage and the pestilence and the stink. It's no longer an environment fit for humans. The city is sick.

That's what would happen inside our bodies if our detoxification systems went on strike. In fact, a version of that nightmare is exactly what does happen. And while it has nothing to do with putting good things—like nutrients, oxygen, or water—into our bodies, detoxification is a life force just as important as the others.

Nowadays, when people talk about detox, they usually mean cleaning up after bad habits (like alcohol, tobacco, or recreational drugs) and man-made poisons (like pollution and industrial chemicals) that collect inside us.

But our bodies know only that there are things—lots of things—

that need to be thrown out. It is our detox system's job to do just that—to take out the trash. All of it, natural and man-made.

For instance, every time we inhale, we extract oxygen from the air. The rest is residue, like car exhaust. And so we exhale, and blow out the carbon, nitrogen, and other gases and toxins that would poison us. Every exhalation, from birth until death, is the detox system at work. Our lungs are an important part of the process.

Our skin is our first line of defense against external threats, acting as a barrier to germs and poisons. Sweat's main job is to control our temperature. But it too is part of the detox system, transporting urea and excess salt and other minerals out of our bodies through the pores. It also carries away bacteria and viruses that collect on the skin.

Our lymphatic system transports white blood cells and other immune system cells made in the thymus gland and bone marrow throughout the body, and then returns with toxins and carcinogens to the lymph nodes, where they can be filtered and destroyed.

But our livers and kidneys are the main organs of the detox system. They have a lot to handle.

We eat. Even good, healthy things. Our bodies break the food down into thousands of components, and then determine what to absorb and where to send it. This is yet another miracle that takes place continually inside our bodies. We instantly recognize, at the cellular level, what we can use and what we can't, and then we transport everything where it belongs.

But a lot in our food doesn't get absorbed. It has to go out in the trash. Even wholesome, life-affirming vegetables and fruits contain toxins. It's how the plants discourage creatures (like us) who would otherwise feed on them to excess. Caffeine is a natural insecticide. If you mix coffee grounds into soil, most critters take off. These natural toxins are just as powerful as any man-made ones. Thanks to evolution, for instance, there's a variety of plant that contains a chemical that works like insect birth control.

Prussic acid found in apples, prunes, and peaches can, in high amounts, impair our use of oxygen. Goitrogens contained in cruciferous vegetables can interfere with thyroid function. The FDA doesn't regulate these natural toxins. It's up to us to handle them.

The useful parts of our food make their way into our blood and then to our cells, but even that's not the end of the journey. Nutrients enter the cells, where energy is created. But all energy produces waste—think smoke and ash from burning coal or oil. The residue must be removed from inside our cells so they can function properly. Considering that we have more than 70 trillion cells, this accounts for a lot of trash—70 trillion trash cans to be continually emptied. The debris passes through the cell membranes and is transported to our kidneys and liver. There, waste is filtered and dispatched to the bladder and colon, which send the toxins on their way. (After which they are recycled by nature and eventually reenter our bodies, but that's another conversation.)

And we're constantly creating brand-new cells, so old ones must die to make space. Those dead cells must be carried off and out of our bodies. We replace all of our cells every decade or so, and some are regenerated much faster than that. Cells lining the intestines last less than a week. Our skin gets resurfaced every two weeks, more or less. We grow a new liver every year.

That's a lot of rebuilding. A lot of old cells to flush. And a lot of replication work for our DNA, which sometimes develops mutations along the way. The more stress that DNA is under, the greater the chance for unhealthy mutations, like the kind that cause cancer. Another reason we want to keep our immune systems in good condition.

There's lots of other stuff that we need to toss—bacteria, viruses, a long list of naturally occurring metabolic wastes that we must dispose of lest they hamper our various bodily systems. Off it all goes.

So much creation and transformation goes on inside our bodies. Naturally, there must be an equal amount of cleanup. And so there is, a constant flow in and out, our contents changing all the time.

If all we had to contend with was the waste from good food,

air, and water, we'd be in decent shape. If we eat a healthy diet, with lots of vegetables and fruit, our food will keep us alkaline and high in natural oxygen, vitamins, minerals, phytonutrients, and antioxidants, all of which support the detox process and slow telomere loss, the measureable speed of aging of our DNA. Our overall inflammation level would be manageable.

But no!

There's more stuff. Really bad stuff.

Free radicals, for instance. These are atoms or molecules containing an odd number of electrons, meaning they need to steal one from another atom to stabilize themselves. If free radicals accumulate and create oxidative stress, they cause cell mutations, which can be carcinogenic. They also weaken us by wiping out cytokines, the pathways that our immune system uses to communicate and coordinate its efforts. This is how our bodies know where to send cells to fight off invaders. Damage to those pathways impairs the system's ability to respond.

Free radicals are behind a long list of the modern age's scourges, like heart disease, cancer, autoimmune disorders, arthritis, Alzheimer's, Parkinson's disease, cystic fibrosis, and more.

Free radicals are sometimes created by normal metabolism. Other times they are a result of environmental toxins. Even the oxidative stress caused by intense exercise increases their number. A certain level of free radicals is necessary for breaking down nutrients. Too many, and we're out of balance.

But our bodies are built to handle even free radicals—as long as our detox systems aren't being asked to do more than they can manage.

It's the other, unnatural stuff we take in that is posing the extra threat today. Those bad habits we mentioned, like alcohol and drugs, plus heavy metals, petrochemicals, car exhaust, pesticides, herbicides, miscellaneous inorganic pollutants—that's the kind of trash that hangs around inside our bodies, unmetabolized. These foreign substances, if not expelled, can lodge in our fat, muscle, bone, cartilage, and other tissue. There, over the

course of decades, they linger, gradually poisoning us and inter-
fering with normal bodily functions. Even low-level exposure to
metals such as arsenic, mercury, lead, and cadmium will eventually interfere with our ability to nourish and detoxify ourselves.

The scientific term for any substance that is foreign to our
bodies is *xenobiotic*. Virtually all food that has been packaged,
bottled, or otherwise processed contains some xenobiotic substance. It could be a partially hydrogenated fat, which sounds like
food but is actually a laboratory creation. Maybe it's dye. Maybe it's
artificial flavoring, or some preservative added to keep the food
fresh-seeming far beyond what nature intended. Maybe it's just
something to keep it crunchy or perky on the plate.

Just because we find something on the food shelves of the supermarket doesn't mean our bodies recognize it as food. Two million years of evolution haven't prepared us to adapt to the junk
that's been shoved into food over the past four or five decades. New
additives are being invented and introduced every day. Can anybody seriously believe that they have all been proven safe over the
long term? No, and it's too impractical even to ask. So we cross our
fingers and ingest these substances, not knowing how much we're
getting, or how harmful they might be, or how they might interact
with all the rest of the toxic load we're taking in through our lungs
and our bellies and our skins.

We have created an entirely new habitat, one not designed to
support human health. And now we have to live in it. We're constantly barraged by toxic substances and forces of one kind or
another. The unnatural world outflanks the natural one, and
overwhelms it at every turn.

Columbia University's School of Public Health released a study
estimating that 95 percent of cancers are a result of either diet,
smoking, exposure to the sun, or environmental toxicity. According to the study, more than three thousand chemicals are added
to the food we eat, and more than ten thousand chemical solvents,
emulsifiers, and preservatives are used to process foods.

At birth we already contain a heavy load of toxins and pollutants. In a study done by the Environmental Working Group, two hundred industrial chemicals and pollutants were found in umbilical cord blood taken from randomly selected babies born in US hospitals. Tests revealed pesticides and wastes from burning coal, gasoline, and garbage—substances known to cause cancer, birth defects, and abnormal development.

Dioxin, for example, is perhaps the most toxic substance known to science. It is a class of chemicals unto itself, totally man-made, the by-product of manufacturing processes that involve chloride. Around thirty of the more than four hundred forms of dioxins are considered to have significant toxicity. Dioxins are in the air, in the water, in products we all use and consume every day. They are powerful carcinogens that also impair the immune system and cause fetal developmental problems during pregnancy. It's a nightmare.

According to the World Health Organization, we're getting 90 percent of our exposure to dioxins from food. These chemicals typically embed themselves in fat, which means, of course, that we get them mostly when we eat animal products—meat, dairy, eggs. We shouldn't feel safer eating fish, either; these are a huge repository of dioxins that find their way into the water.

Our detox systems weren't meant to handle dioxins. But they try.

Another common industrial toxin our bodies deal with daily are phthalates, a group of chemicals used to make plastics more flexible and harder to break. They are used in hundreds of products, such as vinyl flooring, adhesives, detergents, lubricating oils, clothes, and personal-care products such as soap, shampoo, hair spray, and nail polish.

A study done for the US Environmental Protection Agency by researchers from the University of Texas School of Public Health found that "phthalates are widely present in U.S. foods," and while intake of individual examples were below the EPA's limits, "cumulative exposure to phthalates is of concern."

Genetically modified organisms are a new breed of toxin—

one of the most gnarly, because they masquerade as plant-based foods. The genetic modification destroys the DNA of the plant cells and re-creates it, replacing something so natural with one of the most unnatural things imaginable. To put pesticides inside the seed of a plant, they have to break open the cells and inject new genes. Maybe this does kill insects—but that means it kills life. We may not like bugs, but their presence means that life is being supported. If something can kill them, do we really think it's healthy for us? Think of all those pesticides the exterminator uses in your house. Do you love the idea of being exposed to deadly poison?

In "Life Force Number One: Nutrition," we discussed the evidence against GMOs. If you want to know still more, read *Seeds of Deception*, a great book by Jeffrey Smith, or watch *Genetic Roulette*, a documentary Smith directed.

We could go on and on listing the evil junk our immune systems have to defend us from every minute of every day, but you get the point: it's bad out there.

Even our emotional lives and interactions with others bring us into situations with a physiologically toxic effect on our bodies. Mental stress, as we discussed, makes us more acidic. Stress also causes changes in our brain chemistry, which lead to inflammation, weakening our immune systems as a result.

We're perfectly able to handle mental as well as physical stress—as long as it is of short duration. But when these stresses are constant, our response to them creates a chronic condition. Robert M. Sapolsky, in a paper called "Why Zebras Don't Get Ulcers," did an analysis of thirty years' worth of research into this. He concluded, "Stress-related disease emerges, predominantly, out of the fact that we so often activate a physiological system that has evolved for responding to acute physical emergencies, but we turn it on for months on end, worrying about mortgages, relationships, and promotions."

Even invisible pollutants—electromagnetic radiation, microwaves, Wi-Fi, cell phone radiation—take their toll.

The cancer rate is rising, despite all our drugs to combat it and knowledge of how to prevent it. Do we really believe this has nothing to do with our overwhelmed detox systems? It's not that there's one new devastatingly toxic chemical or substance that's going to kill us. The EPA and other agencies are always on the lookout for something really and truly deadly. But nobody pays attention to the constant drip of small doses of all the everyday forms of toxicity. At some point the bucket becomes full and begins to spill over. We can handle just so much before one thing finally pushes us over the line.

Remember that scene I described when the trash collectors go on strike and the city is engulfed by garbage? It happens that way inside our own skins. Over the course of decades, the toxins accumulate. Our livers and kidneys and lungs can no longer keep up. Inflammation is how our bodies protect themselves from disease and injury, but if it goes on too long, inflammation can itself be harmful.

It's a perfect example of what happens after our immune systems become overtaxed. The inflammatory response is meant to protect us from short-term threats, like infections or injuries. But continual assaults put us in a constant state of inflammation. Our bodies can't take it forever.

The liver is responsible for around five hundred different actions that we know of, and supports virtually every organ in the body. It is the mainstay of our detox system—virtually everything we ingest passes through it. Literally like a filter, it picks toxins out of our bloodstream, neutralizes them, and sends them to the exits.

It is such a hardy organ that it's difficult to damage, and even then it alone is able to regenerate itself. But bad diet, obesity, too much alcohol, environmental toxins, and improperly metabolized prescription drugs can cause a condition known as fatty liver. This can impair the organ's ability to detoxify our blood. The fat deposits give toxins a place to hide.

Our kidneys, too, can be damaged by the bad habits they are

meant to protect us from. Researchers at Johns Hopkins University followed more than two thousand young adults for fifteen years. The ones who were obese or ate diets high in red meat, processed foods, and sugary drinks were dramatically more likely to develop a condition known as proteinuria—protein in the urine, a sign of kidney damage—than those who had healthy dietary and lifestyle habits.

The more toxic our world becomes, the greater our kidneys' burden—and then we make matters worse by the way we eat, drink, and live. Today, kidney disease kills more Americans than breast and prostate cancer combined. But for some reason we don't spend much time worrying about our poor overworked kidneys.

More than 10 percent of Americans have chronic kidney disease, but many of us don't even know it; the condition shows no symptoms. Although there is a urine test for protein, most people don't discover they have kidney disease until it's so far along that they need dialysis. High blood pressure raises the risk even more—one-fifth of people with hypertension also have kidney disease.

Kidneys do more than filter toxins. They help maintain our acid-alkaline balance and our electrolytes, regulate blood pressure, and stimulate red blood cell production. But even these functions are necessary to support our detox systems. If our kidneys are impaired, they can't do any of their jobs properly. Our immunity suffers. Next, something bad strikes us out of the blue. Really? In fact we set the stage for it, perhaps over the course of decades.

Our detox systems now have to handle too much. In time we become slightly more vulnerable to external threats. Our immune systems falter just enough. That's when a carcinogen we once neutralized with ease suddenly begins to alter how our genes express themselves.

# The Foundation of Our Detox System

As we've already said, an awful lot of the human body is devoted
to protecting us from serious harm: skin, sweat glands, lungs,
liver, kidneys, bone marrow, thymus, lymphatic system, immune
system, intestinal microbes, bladder, and colon.

Of course, that's not what's really keeping us safe.

None of those amazing organs and marvelous systems would
work very well if not for the other four life forces. Nutrition, hydration, oxygenation, and alkalization are the true foundation of
our detox system, the real underpinning of our immunity from
disease.

If we don't keep those four things right, we're dead ducks. Our
bodies will become like that street I described, buried under garbage and filth.

This is the most important thing to remember about our ability
to heal ourselves: a strong, healthy, well-fed body is an unfriendly
environment for disease. I can't emphasize this enough. Every illness, impairment, disorder, and deficiency damages our immune
system's ability to function. The first step to efficient detoxification is to take care of everything else. If we promote the good
things and prevent the bad, we allow our bodies to be the strong,
disease-fighting machines they are meant to be.

If we do that, we won't need to worry about "catching" a cold.
That term is one of my pet peeves; it indicates a total misunder-
standing of how we become sick. I'm going to use a slightly disgusting image to make my point: if someone with the flu were to
sneeze right in my face, right in my open mouth, and my immune
system were strong and functioning, I would inhale plenty
of germs, but not one of them would sicken me. That's because
my healthy internal environment would be too strong to penetrate.

If we are run down and vulnerable, however—if we are acidic, dehydrated, oxygen-poor, and lacking the right nutrients—we offer harmful bacteria, viruses, and even carcinogens a welcoming home. And they're happy to take advantage of our hospitality.

That's the true mechanism of illness: we don't catch the cold, we create the conditions through our tendencies—food, habits, stress—to either welcome or repel the illness. Same for heart disease, cancer, stroke—the top causes of death today. In many instances, they are associated with unhealthy behaviors. Whether we're aware of it or not, sickness is often a result of a choice we made. Mosquitoes don't show up unless there is stagnant water, a place where they can multiply and thrive. The same goes for microscopic bugs, the sources of our colds and diseases. What kind of environment are we creating?

Of course, sometimes there are circumstances totally beyond our control. If a child becomes sick, he or she didn't make the lifestyle choices that contributed to the disease. Even adults living healthy lifestyles become ill with chronic diseases. This just underscores the need to make conscious choices about what to eat and not eat, how much activity to get, whether or not to endure stress and toxic relationships.

Remember, somewhere between 10 and 20 percent of disease is caused purely by genetic disposition, and the rest is strongly influenced by lifestyle choices. We carry many genes, but they don't all express themselves. The DNA listens to the environment that we create. Unhealthy diet and other bad habits promote one kind of genetic expression. Eating good, fresh plant foods and getting plenty of water and exercise encourage another.

Nutrition is the single most important factor in the functioning of the immune .

This is why, in the Third World, malnutrition, insufficient clean water, overcrowding, and lack of sanitation make infection a common cause of serious illness and death. It's why in India, as we discussed earlier, the spice turmeric is so beloved. Indians eat it every day. It's what gives curry its yellow color. There's another reason it's so popular: turmeric contains curcumin, a powerful anti-inflammatory and immune booster. Food and spices are the poor person's pharmacy.

Fortunately for us, we can take advantage of science's miraculous medicines. But, as happens so often, the solution becomes the problem—only worse. Once people often died from bacteria that their immune systems couldn't handle; then antibiotics were discovered. The first clue to possible trouble was there in the name: *Biotic* signifies life; an antibiotic kills life. Who could foresee a reason to worry?

Flash forward to now, when 70 to 80 percent of all antibiotics administered in the United States are given to animals. These drugs are no longer used just to fight disease—they make livestock grow bigger and keep the beasts healthy enough to eat. The overuse of antibiotics promoted the rise of drug-resistant bacteria, which now kill more than 100,000 Americans a year. Even indirectly, meat harms us.

In addition to overall good nutrition, our immune systems specifically need zinc, iodine, the B vitamins (especially $B_6$ and $B_{12}$), vitamins A, C, and E, iron, copper, folic acid, and the antioxidant coenzyme $Q_{10}$. Zinc supports the thymus, which creates the T-cells that fight infection. The mineral selenium also helps our bodies make T cells. Glutathione is known as the "master antioxidant," meaning it does more to fight free radicals than any other known substance. Carotenoids—pigmented nutrients that give fruits and vegetables their bright colors—also contain antioxidants, as does tea, especially green tea.

All these substances can be found in dietary supplements. But whole foods are still the best, most efficient source. Zinc is contained in peanuts, dark chocolate, toasted wheat germ, and roasted pumpkin and squash seeds. (It's also found in oysters, liver, and crab.) Research published in the *American Journal of Clinical Nutrition* showed that we can get all the selenium we need by eating just two Brazil nuts a day. We can also get it from sunflower seeds, mushrooms, whole grains, and onions.

Antioxidants are the group of vitamins, minerals, and other nutrients that fight the oxidation created by free radicals. They can prevent mutation of the gene p53, for instance, which suppresses tumors. Antioxidants also protect our DNA, which is another way of preventing cancer from finding a hospitable environment inside our bodies.

Fiber is particularly important to the detox process, both the soluble kind our bodies absorb and use and the insoluble kind that just passes through our gut (and cleans the passage of toxins along the way). That's another good reason for eating whole fruits, vegetables, and grains.

And we need to drink a lot of water. Water is an extremely powerful detoxification agent in our bodies. If we are properly hydrated, we have the best means of transporting toxins and other debris to the exits.

Dehydration actually hinders the immune system in several ways. First, it causes histamine production in the body to increase, which also triggers the production of a chemical called vasopressin, a strong suppressor of the immune system. Excess histamine also causes the shutdown of interferon, a critical anti-cancer chemical that is present in a hydrated body. Finally, histamine suppresses immune activity in the bone marrow, which is the central production center of the white blood cells— which can destroy and digest cancer cells.

Of course our water should be as clean as possible, since waterborne toxins and irritants only add to our burden. City water is usually treated with chloride to kill potentially harmful bacteria. This is a good thing—except that then we end up having to deal with the chloride, fluoride, pharmaceuticals, and high amounts of total dissolved solids in the water, all of which pose their own health hazards. Better if we can find a safe, untreated source of water.

Even physical activity plays a part in detox. As we said earlier, excessively hard workouts actually increase the number of free radicals. They're caused by consuming oxygen, after all. Tests show that ultramarathoners and those who do intense exercise actually experience damage to their DNA as a result.

This damage can be blocked in advance, however, by eating foods rich in antioxidants. Researchers from the Biomedicine and Sport Science Research Group, Edinburgh Napier University, tested the effect of watercress on exercise-induced oxidation. Subjects who ate it before they worked out actually had lower levels of free radicals afterward. Those who didn't eat it had the opposite result—more potential DNA damage. The scientists also dripped watercress directly onto blood loaded up with free radicals, and found the same effect: the vegetable cleansed the blood.

In another study, this one published in the *American Journal of Clinical Nutrition*, researchers found that watercress was able to reduce DNA damage by 17 percent. "The results," the authors wrote, "support the theory that consumption of watercress can be linked to a reduced risk of cancer via decreased damage to DNA and possible modulation of antioxidant status by increasing carotenoid concentrations."

More often, exercise has a beneficial effect on our detox systems. The more we sweat, the more we drink, and the more we urinate, which flushes toxins from our bodies. Toxins like dioxins are stored in fat cells, and so the fitter we are, the fewer places for poisons to linger. If we're out of shape, we're probably eating an unhealthy diet, which itself is a drag on our immune systems.

Finally, we need to become aware of all the toxins in our environments and do our best to avoid exposure. That can be a challenge. We're into physical contact with the world twenty-four hours a day, and whatever we touch, touches us. It all leaves a residue—on our skin, in our mouths, our lungs, our cells.

Every day new chemical substances are introduced into the world. They're in the air we breathe and the water we drink, in the lumber used to build our houses and the furniture and carpets that fill them. In our clothing. In our soap and shampoo and deodorant and perfume and laundry detergent—any personal care product that has a fragrance contains irritants that our bodies then have to neutralize. They exist in nearly every man-made object we touch. We unknowingly absorb something from all of it. Researchers find scores of these substances in normal, healthy human beings—heavy metals, even uranium. The onslaught is constant. Just read the ingredients of your deodorant or moisturizer or body wash. Not many natural substances in there.

What can we do about this portion of our toxic load? Take control. Make better choices. Try hard to limit our physical exposure to chemical badness. Keep in mind that it's not just where food is concerned that we need to be vigilant; if something touches us, it feeds us, whether we want it to or not. Some people buy only environmentally friendly personal and household products because they care about their impact on the planet. But it goes way beyond that. If something is bad for Earth, it's probably not so great for us, either. Don't support companies that don't care about you.

How can we know if our detox system is being overburdened? All the little things that seem to afflict a lot of people—more like minor complaints and irritations than anything serious, or so we fool ourselves. Dry skin, acne, headaches. Itchy eyes. Indigestion. Constipation. Achy joints. Fatigue. All these are caused by irritants and inflammations that are getting the better of us. The signs are so diverse and so subtle that we don't associate them with any particular cause. That's what makes them so dangerous. We don't recognize them as the early warning signals of something possibly serious. We need to know what to look for if we're going to do something about it.

# Simple To-Do List ✓

- Take care of the other four life forces—proper nutrition, hydration, oxygenation, and alkalization—in order to boost your detox system. Otherwise, you can't expect your body to fight off disease and rid you of the harmful substances you inadvertently take in.

- Don't become a boozehound or a drug user. But even so, modern life hits us with so much air and water pollution, so many unknown chemicals in our food and drink, such an array of industrial additives and irritants in our clothing, personal care products and surroundings, that we have to take care to avoid these harmful substances as well when possible.

- Eat foods and adopt habits that support your liver and kidney function, since those organs (especially the liver) have to handle all the toxicity that you absorb every day.

- Get plenty of iron, copper, zinc, folic acid, and the co-enzyme $Q_{10}$, as well as the vitamins A, B (especially $B_6$ and $B_{12}$), C and E, so that your immune system can function properly. Brightly colored fruits and vegetables are typically high in antioxidants, which is why it's important to let your eyes guide you.

# How to Feed the Kids

Here's something I see all the time.

People are making positive changes in what they eat and don't eat. And it shows. Great!

Then it comes time to feed the kids—and all those good intentions and smart decisions go out the window. In theory, every parent wants what's best for his or her children. But for some reason, that doesn't always extend to what they eat and drink. It's bad enough when the parents eat lousy food too. It's even worse when parents who know the importance of good nutrition still let their kids eat badly. It's like quitting cigarettes but allowing your children to smoke.

Despite some recent improvement, we're still facing unacceptably high obesity and diabetes among children. We claim to view that as a national emergency. The most recent study in the news claims that one-fifth of American teenage boys suffer from attention deficit and hyperactivity disorder. And it's not just them—girls have it, too. Another worrisome development.

These kids are nutrient-deprived, sleep-deprived, dehydrated, and loaded with toxic chemicals, and then we're shocked to learn that they're paying the price? It would be shocking if they weren't.

I mentioned elsewhere the development of two distinct food cultures today, one good, the other bad. There's been another division, too—one food culture for adults, another for children. At restaurants, two separate menus. For adults, healthy choices, a variety of vegetables and salads, spices and flavors, freshly made in the kitchen. Beautiful meals. On the kids' menu, there's pizza, white-flour pasta, low-quality chicken that's processed, cut into cute shapes, and then breaded and deep fried, hot dogs, hamburgers, sodas, chocolate milk—all the usual suspects. The message to children is clear: these are the things we expect you to choose. Feel free to ignore the real food.

It's not just the restaurants. Each food culture has its own source of information, too. Kid food media consists of commercials for sugary cereal and Happy Meals and soft drinks. Youngsters listen avidly when their peers debate the quality of this cheap stuffed pizza over that one, or the new frozen yogurt parlor where you shovel in your own choice of candy toppings. The messages are all around them, like air. They don't read newspaper stories about the latest health research, or watch the medical TV shows. They're checking their friends' tweets about the new fast-food joint or looking at their Instagram photos of today's feast. When kids get hungry, they aren't thinking about their cholesterol. They're not worried about salt or sugar or fat, let alone disease and infirmity and mortality.

Of course parents are expected to know better. We take our children for annual checkups and consult the pediatrician at the first sign of something wrong. We buy them the best car seats on the market, and research the finest schools and camps. Our devotion to our children's future well-being is boundless. And still we let them dump whatever garbage they like into their bellies. Sure, you wish she'd eat the same organic arugula salad you're having, but if she won't? Bring on the french fries. Who wants to hear complaining all through dinner? And it would be great if he'd choose water instead of that sweet sports drink. But better he drinks that than nothing at all, right?

Once upon a time, when I was small, it probably made sense to give kids a cookie or piece of candy or ice cream cone as a treat. Back then, eating a little junk was a special event. Even a young body could handle it. Children weren't assaulting their systems with a continuous stream of sugar, salt, unhealthy fats, and chemicals from food manufacturing processes that didn't yet exist.

Not so long ago, children ate the same things their parents did—whole foods, made from scratch at home, served at the table. The idea that adults and children eat differently would have seemed absurd. Once the single food culture split into two, along came childhood obesity. Think it's a coincidence?

My own path to good nutrition started when I was a kid. I didn't really know what I was doing, only that I felt lousy and somebody said that eating differently could change me. That's all it took. It's probably true that you can't force a child to adopt good habits. But if we act as though we expect them to eat unhealthy things, they don't stand a chance.

Even the healthiest of our kids are in danger. High school and college athletes inhabit these amazing bodies, and they work them until they are strong and fast and beautiful inside and out. And then as soon as practice ends or the game is over, they stampede the nearest McDonald's or Burger King or pizzeria. And they start their days with Dunkin' Donuts and Red Bull. It's not easy to convince them that if they ate and drank better, they'd be even healthier and stronger. But it's true. And they're acquiring bad habits that will take years for their bodies to unlearn—if ever.

I wish I could convince those kids that if they eat lousy food today, they are incurring a nutritional debt that someday they will have to pay.

I want to tell them they can eat processed junk and soda and all the rest now and never feel a thing. Then, when they turn forty or fifty or sixty, the bill for all that nutritional debt they piled up over the decades will come due. Suddenly their bodies will be limited because of choices they made when they were young and immortal. Maybe it will be diabetes, or heart disease, or back trouble, or painful joints, or hypertension.

And they'll ask themselves the question everybody asks at that painful moment: Why me? But we adults know why.

We're sending kids the message that their youth somehow protects them from the ill effects of poor nutrition—as though being young is a form of immunity. But it isn't. Real damage is being done to kids' bodies when they eat and drink the wrong things. Our two biggest killers, heart disease and cancer, take decades to develop. They may start in childhood. And yet some of us just shrug our shoulders and let our children indulge their tastes for junk foods and sugary everything. Someday, when those kids grow up and become ill, will we make the connection to the high-risk behavior of their youth? New science is already linking childhood nutrition to adult health. You can bet you will be hearing more about it going forward.

We let children make bad choices about something as important as nutrition, but we wouldn't let them make similar decisions about other things. Kids will innocently eat garbage, just like they will spend all their time playing video games or staying up late watching junk TV. But we don't let them do that, do we? We take pride in ourselves as parents for insisting that they study and sleep. So why fill them up with bad food and toxins?

Maybe it's true that kids need to find their own way and decide to eat right and move and be healthy. Maybe we should let them say, *I'm gaining weight and looking sloppy, and I don't like it. I can change it. I am in control of myself.*

But we still need to steer them better than we're doing. Be the change for yourself, and your children will be more likely to notice the respect and love you have for your body and apply them to themselves.

# Simple To-Do List

- Don't let your kids eat or drink anything that you wouldn't consume. Can it be any simpler than that? Children are developing lifelong habits and tastes now. It's a mistake to think that because they're young they have some special immunity from lousy nutrition.

- Make your kids drink plenty of water. Typical children dislike drinking water only because they've been offered so many sweet, brightly colored, bubbly alternatives in fancy packaging. Can we blame them for refusing boring old water? Researchers are finding links between insufficient water and ADD and hyperactivity. What if those kids would have benefitted instead from simply drinking more? Before we let our children become drug consumers, we ought to try improving their diet and drinking habits first.

- Help your teenagers understand that the food choices they make today may have a huge impact on their health in the future. As science has shown us, chronic diseases such as heart disease and cancer begin developing when we're young.

# How to Supplement

*The Role and Use of*
*Nutritional Supplements*

L et's start by reminding ourselves of something important: supplementation is not replacement.

We can only be healthy if first we eat and drink properly, and get as much nutrition as possible from fresh, whole foods. We can't keep our bad habits and then think we'll make up for it by swallowing pills. Fact is, our bodies won't even be able to use those nutritional supplements very well if we're not already eating well and taking care of ourselves. We need to lose that big-fix mentality.

Still, unless we live on organic farms far from the polluted world, and eat an insanely wide variety of fresh-from-the-ground whole foods, mostly uncooked, we will probably need to supplement our diets with things we'd otherwise lack. It would be wonderful if that weren't the case, but let's be real.

If our food isn't providing enough of a particular nutrient or protective substance, we should turn first to my passion—superfoods. ("My Life as a Superfood Hunter" is devoted to this subject.) Superfoods are whole foods, same as any other. We eat them unadulterated, as they are found in nature, except sometimes dried or powdered. Superfoods are extremely nutrient-dense and usually somewhat exotic, at least to us. They are meant to fill in the gaps in our normal nutritional profile.

When we need more vitamin C, for instance, we don't have to take a pill. We can try introducing some powdered moringa leaves, camu camu, or goji berries into our diet, and that should do the trick—without having to resort to something created in a lab or factory.

But even a healthy diet of food and superfood isn't enough. We need a little extra.

The only questions are: What do we supplement, and how?

# Vitamins

OK, let's start with the basics. We should try to get virtually *all* our vitamins and minerals from what we eat and drink. True, we can find pills and capsules containing synthesized versions of just about every nutrient there is. But then we are getting just one thing, whereas the fruit or vegetable contains many of them, thousands— vitamins and minerals, plus antioxidants, enzymes, phytonutri- ents, cofactors, and more, all with very specific biological effects on our bodies, in a symphony of balance created by nature.

Why do you think virtually all the nutritional supplements and pharmaceutical drugs on the market are inspired by plant chemicals? Because nature has figured some things out better than we ever will. Man can never re-create what nature has al- ready created—period. There are always unintended side effects when we isolate components in a lab. Nature is polymorphic—it has many aspects, outcomes, and benefits.

Anyway, we have no idea, really, what is inside that jar or con- tainer of whatever supplement we're considering. Every formula- tion is different. Each contains some version of whatever the label proclaims, but we have no proof that our bodies will find it bio- available, which is what counts most. We're also in the dark about what other substances it contains—and it always contains some- thing else.

When we eat an apple, however, or lettuce, there's no guess-work. We know it's alive, just like we are. We know all the ingredients without having to read the fine print.

I started by saying we should get our vitamins from natural, whole-food sources, but there are two exceptions.

## The Role of Vitamin D in Cancer Prevention

Vitamin D is one of the most powerful cancer-fighting elements in the body, and it possesses countless other beneficial, immune-boosting capabilities. We usually get it from exposure to sun-light. If we're wearing sunblock, however, then we're cutting off our bodies' ability to produce this important vitamin. An SPF of 8 eliminates 99.9 percent of the vitamin D production capacity of the skin—clearly not a good idea. Not to mention that most sun-screens contain the chemical oxybenzone, which may disrupt the hormone system and irritate the skin. There are so-called experts today who advise people to wear sunblock 100 percent of the time. That's silly. We should take care not to burn, but we shouldn't fear the sun.

Even if we get sunlight, though, we probably need to take a vitamin D supplement—especially if we work indoors, or live where winters are truly cold. According to a 2006 survey of existing research, published in the *American Journal of Public Health*, "The majority of studies found a protective relationship between sufficient vitamin D status and lower risk of cancer. The evidence suggests that efforts to improve vitamin D status, for example by vitamin D supplementation, could reduce cancer incidence and mortality at low cost, with few or no adverse effects."

Another natural source of vitamin D is mushrooms. Eating them will provide a healthy dose. But there are also supplements made from mushrooms that have been exposed to UVA/UVB light. That's the way to go. It's better than taking vitamin D that has been synthesized in a lab.

### The Role of Vitamin B in Cancer Prevention

The second vitamin we probably need to supplement is $B_{12}$. It's very important for building blood and maintaining the nervous system, along with supporting energy production. Animal foods— meat, dairy, eggs, whey—are the usual source. But that may not be enough, especially if you're trying to eat a mostly plant diet. When we vegans and vegetarians lack it, we can eat fermented foods or take nutritional yeast or vitamin supplements containing methyl $B_{12}$, which is easier to break down than any other form of the vitamin. Ten micrograms of $B_{12}$ spread over a day appears to be a good target.

# Enzymes

Back in "Life Force Number One: Nutrition," we talked a lot about enzymes. It's almost impossible to exaggerate their importance to health, and it's difficult to get enough naturally. After we reach our thirties, enzyme production in the body drops off big-time.

Enzymes are made of amino acids that we either create inside our bodies or get from outside sources. Enzymes are simply catalysts—they make every single biochemical reaction in our bodies happen. Which means that without them, nothing—no creation of energy, no absorption of nutrients, no detoxification of cells—takes place. Life itself would come to a screeching halt were it not for enzymes. They are the labor force of the body. That's pretty important.

Our bodies contain three types of enzyme. The first kind is in whole, fresh foods. These enzymes help our bodies to metabolize the food we eat. But the enzymes die if heated to over 118 degrees Fahrenheit. That's one of the reasons that raw food is important.

Most of us are not going to eat every meal uncooked, though; it would be boring. Cooking is an expression of our humanity. And in some cases, cooking actually makes some food healthier.

A lot of fat-soluble vitamins and other nutrients become more biologically available when heated. Cooked tomatoes provide more lycopene than raw. The vitamin A and carotenoids contained in carrots become more bioavailable when cooked. But keep in mind that a lot of other water-soluble nutrients are destroyed by cooking, including vitamins B and C. So when it comes to vegetables, 75 percent raw is a good goal.

The second type is digestive enzymes. Each of these is devoted to metabolizing a specific nutrient. Amylase breaks down carbohydrates. It exists in our saliva, which is where digestion really begins. Lipase is the enzyme that works on fats. Protease breaks down proteins. There are others that work on fiber, dairy, and so on.

The third kind, systemic or proteolytic enzymes, are catalysts for all biochemical reactions, just like the digestive kind. But these operate throughout our entire bodies. They do a lot of important jobs, such as fighting inflammation, controlling our immune systems, and cleansing our blood, among others. There has been a great deal of research lately into their role in preventing our top two killers, heart disease and cancer. Taking systemic enzyme supplements is one of the best nontoxic ways to eliminate inflammation of all kinds. That's crucial because of how chronic bodywide inflammation damages our overall health.

Researchers have used systemic enzyme supplementation to treat sports injuries. In tests, enzymes were given to boxers and soccer players before they performed, and in both cases they experienced fewer injuries than those who didn't take them. Enzymes are also believed to decrease the time it takes to recover from injuries and promote healing after orthopedic surgery, because they increase blood flow. We can take over-the-counter medications such as aspirin and Tylenol to do the same thing, but these have been found to cause liver damage. That organ has enough to do nowadays, given the toxic level of everyday life. So you can see why it's better if we can handle the job with enzymes instead.

# Probiotics

Probiotics are living bacteria that are beneficial to other living bacteria. As we discussed in "Feeding Our Other Body," our bodies depend heavily on the trillions of bacteria we carry around with us, mostly in our intestines. These single-cell organisms aren't even human, but they help us to break down and utilize what we eat. They perform lots of other important functions, too. We couldn't live without them, and when they are out of balance, we suffer. There are thousands of different kinds, some of which are good for us, some not.

Back at the turn of the twentieth century, the Russian Nobel laureate Ilya Mechnikov theorized that when certain intestinal bacteria digested proteins, they produced toxins that made our internal environment acidic and promoted aging. He theorized that eating fermented dairy—he used sour milk—would introduce microbes that could decrease our intestinal acidity and promote health and longevity. Since then, probiotics have been found to have an anticarcinogenic effect, and to improve ailments like irritable bowel, high cholesterol, hypertension, and even depression.

Only within the past thirty years have we begun to understand how supplementing certain bacteria can benefit our digestive systems, and there's still no definitive scientific "proof" that it works. But I (and plenty of other people) believe in it.

Probiotics are present in cultured foods such as yogurt and kefir, and fermented foods such as kimchi, sauerkraut, miso, natto, and kombucha. You'll notice that those foods aren't a part of what we call the standard American diet. Once, most of the planet's population ate some fermented dishes. People understood then that food's job was to promote internal health. We've lost that sense of nutritional mission, and proof of this is the lack of fermented, probiotic-rich foods in the normal diet. We should all make it a point to eat probiotic-rich foods.

Then, if we still need more, we can find supplements in the refrigerated food section of most health food stores. Look for products containing bifidobacteria or *Lactobacillus*.

They are kept cool because they have to be alive when they reach our intestines.

Lately, a somewhat radical form of supplementation—fecal transplantation—has been used successfully to improve the bacterial environment of the intestines. A small amount of feces from a healthy person is implanted in the gut of someone suffering from intestinal ailments. Instantly, the microbial composition changes for the better.

Yes, that is correct, poop transplants. The really fascinating part is that the transplant recipients immediately express cravings for the foods that the donor favored. Talk about a fast and dirty solution! I am not saying this is the ultimate answer, but it does prove the importance of microbes to who we are.

# Essential Fatty Acids

In nutritional terms, the word *essential* is used to describe substances we need that our bodies don't produce—and that we must thus get from outside sources. Our bodies need fatty acids for a number of important tasks, such as the formation of the cell membranes and tissues of the brain and nervous system. Lipids are key for the creation and maintenance of healthy cells. Just two layers of lipids protect our DNA from damage and help to preserve our telomeres. This protection is composed of fatty acids.

Two of these are essential, which is why we need to get both alpha-linolenic acid (better known as omega-3 fats and oils) and linoleic acid (omega-6) from outside sources. These are contained in leafy greens and seeds, but the richest providers are oily fish like salmon and mackerel and shellfish. We especially need omega-3 fatty acids, to balance out omega-6s, of which we tend to have too much.

Omega-3 fatty acids are anti-inflammatory and fight free radicals. They have been associated with cardiac health. Essential fatty acids also help pull oxygen inside the cell, where it helps protect us from bacteria and viruses. Remember, in "Life Force Number Three: Oxygenation" we discussed the importance of proper cell respiration in keeping cancer away.

As I said, we can get fatty acids from fish, but then we may be creating other problems. People who eat fish regularly need to be tested for mercury in their blood. There are also PCBs, dioxins, and other lethal pollutants found in the water, and so in the fish, too.

That's why the best way to supplement these essential fatty acids may not be the most common one—fish oil capsules. We don't know what those fish ate, or what toxins they absorbed. We have to recognize the world we inhabit. Better to eat chia seeds, flaxseed, sacha inchi oil, and walnuts, and then add in DHA and EPA supplements made from algae rather than fish oil.

# Protein

As we discuss elsewhere in the book, many of us are getting unhealthily high levels of protein due to our love of meat, fish, and eggs. But some of us—especially vegans and vegetarians, who do not always make good food choices—are in danger of getting too little. Remember, simply avoiding animal food doesn't make a person well nourished. We still have to be smart eaters.

For active people, I recommend a vegan protein powder, for a few reasons. One, because it's not made of milk whey, you won't have to worry about whether you can absorb the lactose contained in dairy products. Most people who are lactose-intolerant don't know it. It's also best to avoid exposure to the hormones and other products used to raise cows, or the GMOs used to feed them.

Vegan proteins come from peas, oats, spirulina, chlorella, and other plants. They contain the most important amino acids, such as glutamine, leucine, isoleucine, arginine, and valine, but in a form our bodies can easily absorb. That makes life less stressful for the intestines, which need all the help they can get.

Especially if we exercise with intensity, our bodies need protein to build, repair, and maintain lean muscle mass. Get the powders, not capsules, for best results.

# Sulfur

MSM—methylsulfonylmethane—is a naturally occurring sulfur compound that helps transport nutrients in and out of cells. This alone is a very important job. But we also need sulfur to help us produce glutathione, the master antioxidant. Sulfur has been shown to reduce joint pain and inflammation and to help muscle recovery from exercise. It improves cellular health overall. There hasn't been a lot of discussion of sulfur's role in our health, but that's changing as we come to understand how vital it is.

MSM (which is not related to common sulfur, sulfates, or sulfites) is extremely important for cell permeability and reduces oxidative stress. It is contained in fresh, raw greens, but even if we eat them, we may not be getting enough, for the simple reason that our soil has become depleted of nutrients. That's why I am a great believer in MSM supplementation. But not all MSM is created equal. The proven best results come from MSM processed through the distillation of natural lignans, like the pine tree, and not through chemical extraction.

# Greens

Finally, we all need to get more greens than we do. Of course eating fresh, organic kale, romaine, spinach, dandelion, and arugula is the place to start. Add in some superfoods such as moringa leaves, chlorella, and spirulina, and you're adding a lot more good stuff. Then consider marine phytoplanktons, the mother green from the ocean, the biggest donor of oxygen to Earth. They contain trace minerals, DHA, omega-3s, and other substances that benefit the brain and nervous system. Green foods increase detoxification, balance acidity and alkalinity, lower the inflammatory response, and boost the immune system.

# Simple To-Do List

- Take some essential supplements. Our current nutritional environment is such that we need to take supplements where our diets are lacking. Eat healthy foods and drink plenty of water first, and then support those habits with supplements.

- Take a vitamin D supplement. Most of us don't get enough, and it is so important in cancer prevention. If you're not eating animal foods you should almost certainly take vitamin $B_{12}$, which performs several important functions.

- Take enzyme supplements, which support digestive health and necessary biochemical events that take place throughout our bodies. As we discussed in this chapter, most people should also be taking supplements of certain minerals, essential fatty acids, and even protein (for those of us who don't get it from animal foods).

# A Final Word on the
# Five Life Forces

As I've mentioned before—and more than once—the key thing to remember about the five life forces is that each one you get right works to support the other four. If we eat properly, that good nutrition will automatically keep us slightly alkaline, and that in turn will help keep us mineral-rich. Healthy eating also means we're getting lots of antioxidants, which aid our immune systems in fighting disease. If we eat right and drink enough water, our tissues will be oxygen-rich and fill us with energy. Hydration and oxygenation also help our bodies to eliminate toxins and cellular debris.

The opposite is also true: if we fail to maintain one of the life forces, it drags down the others, setting off a cascade of failures that can be seriously damaging over time. If we eat a lousy diet, our ability to detoxify ourselves is weakened. If we can't detox right, our enyzmatic function is diminished. When that happens, all our cells suffer. Drink too little water and cells can't properly metabolize the foods we eat. When that takes place, we put extra stress on our detox systems. If we're acidic, our cells become oxygen-poor, which gives cancer and other diseases a better chance to defeat our immune systems.

The meaning in all these connections is clear—the five life forces are in reality just five parts of a single life force. This is where all our scientific knowledge suddenly turns into wisdom.

To me, it's mind-blowing—that moment of clarity when we see that we have the power to nourish ourselves, regenerate ourselves, energize ourselves, heal ourselves, truly *know* ourselves. All thanks to air, water, and whole, fresh foods.

Pretty amazing.

# One Last Thing . . .

I lied. There's a sixth life force.

This is the most important one of all, though it's hard to imagine what could matter more than breathing, eating, and drinking.

But without the sixth life force, we'll never gain control over the other five.

The sixth life force is attitude.

My attitude is what has made me so fanatical about my health—and now yours too. I want the best life possible: a SuperLife. And I hope that you will want the same for yourself. We underestimate the force we have as individuals to create and change. We have so much power, if we will just allow ourselves to use it.

My attitude is what has made me so obsessive about finding the best food there is, the freshest, cleanest, most potent nutrition the planet has to offer. For some reason I can never get to the point where I say, "OK, this is good enough." I'm always aware that there's a higher level, some new thing I can't even imagine right now, and if I search, maybe I'll find it. Even if I don't get there, I want to try.

I have traveled hundreds of thousands of miles in the process, bumping into very old cultures, natural healers, and traditional ways, and I love doing that. However, it doesn't mean anything unless I apply what I learn and share it—paying it forward, completing the loop.

Attitude is what engages me and pushes me to insist that we are meant to be strong and completely, amazingly alive, and that we owe it to ourselves to do everything possible to get there. It really does drive me a little crazy to see people settle for less than they deserve, especially from themselves. I truly believe that once we recognize the miracle that we possess—the miracle that we *are*—we will all begin to live accordingly.

I've seen the other side of this, too. I think of my father before he died of alcoholism. He was a wonderful man, but he created his world in a way that left him feeling as though he had no choice but to drink. You decide that something is true, and guess what? It is.

Having a great attitude—living the life we want, or at least going for it by taking real action—bestows upon us some practical benefits. We are subject to magnetic forces like everything else on the planet, and it seems that like attracts like. Your positive attitude and actions will draw you toward people who share that outlook, and they will echo and support your efforts to live well. We all give off energy—scientists are actually measuring this now, and studying its effects. Emotions and mood have a powerful influence over our physical beings. That we know for sure.

Still, I didn't study all this health stuff just so I could be smart about something, or so I could tell other people what to do. I learned it because I desired to figure out how to make myself stronger, healthier, and ultimately happy and balanced. It goes back to that day when I was a kid who decided to eat a lot of grapefruit and take control over my body and my life. Since then, all I've wanted was to understand what I have to do to get the most out of living, all the joy and pleasure possible—and then to go do it.

Because as far as I know, I'm not getting another life. If this one doesn't go so well because I didn't make the most of it, too bad. I don't get a do-over.

If you were to go on vacation somewhere, to Paris or even Disney World, you'd want to make the most of the experience—to have the best stay possible. How can you accept any less from your time on this planet?

The main thing to remember is why we're doing this. It's not just to make ourselves healthy. Taking care of the five life forces isn't the point. Learning how to keep our bodies in great shape isn't the ultimate goal. Being healthy matters only because we need good health to have everything else we want: fantastic lives—happy, positive, balanced, full of passion and energy and love. Truly living!

That's what matters most, isn't it?

# Part Two

# The Really Useful Section

Now that we've covered the science of healthy eating and drinking, it's time for the nuts and bolts—putting all that information to good use.

First, I'll go over some of the rules of healthy eating, followed by advice for a kitchen purge. After that, you'll find lists of the foods that contain all the nutrients we need, and then a ten-day eating plan to get you started. Finally I'll share some recipes for those meals, and then I'll leave you with one last to-do list.

# How to Eat

**H**ere's the first rule of healthy eating: We should eat only things we love.

Here's the second rule: We should only love things that are good for us.

There may be a little mental work required in there. Many of us love chocolate chip cookies. And Cheetos. And hot dogs. M&Ms. Frozen burritos. Pepperoni pizza. Jelly doughnuts. Deviled eggs. Twinkies. Big Macs. Beer. Thick, charred steaks. The list goes on . . .

A lot of people love heroin, too, but we don't all allow ourselves to indulge. We understand that as tasty as it may be, it's not worth the damage it will do to us. And so we steer clear.

We need to understand that unhealthy food can be just as damaging as drugs. More, when you think of how many people are hooked on lousy eating. Junk food isn't illegal or frowned upon by society. And it isn't addictive, exactly. But if we eat enough, it can do us plenty of harm.

Junk food is like a bad boyfriend: we love it, but it hurts us.

Tell me this: How can anybody not love a big, ripe, red strawberry? The way it explodes on your tongue with all that sweetness and flavor and juice? Really, can an M&M compare with that? It's as easy to love good food as it is to love bad. Easier. But maybe it requires a little effort at first. We had to learn to love bad food, and so it may take us some time to teach ourselves to love good food instead.

I've said this over and over: eating should be a thrill. Every meal should fill us with happiness. If it doesn't, we're doing something unnatural. We're cheating ourselves out of life's most dependable joy. Too many of our meals today are consumed in a rushed, thoughtless way. We fail to connect what we eat with who we are. That's a big part of our current nutritional crisis, I really believe.

Our senses will guide us if we let them. Eat things that smell good. Raw foods especially send out olfactory signals to what they contain, and our sense of smell can read those messages. We have to pay attention.

The food companies use our olfactory sense against us by engineering products that will appeal to our primal love of certain nutrients, like fat, salt, or sugar. But if you're responding favorably to the scent of a ripe pineapple, or some asparagus, or the perfume of fresh basil on a tomato, it's because your body is trying to tell you something: *Eat this!* Your body intuits what those foods contain, even if you do not. Same with colors—we're visually attracted to the ripe red of cherries, beets, peppers, watermelon, and cranberries without thinking that the color comes from flavonoids, which signal us that antioxidants are present. Or we're drawn to the lush beauty of dark green leaves like spinach, arugula, chard, because our bodies desire food that cleanses our blood and provides valuable minerals.

That's the first basis for choosing what to eat—pure physical desire. Don't eat anything because you *should*. Eat it because you want it, deeply want it! Allow your body to express its most elemental wishes in an authentic way. *Feed me*, comes the call, and our job is to answer it.

How can eating bring us joy if we're sitting there chewing on something we hate? How much care will we devote to shopping and preparing and cooking if we dread the end result? And—most important—how long will it be before we slip back into bad old habits?

As we eat, we need to remember that our food will soon be a part of us. It will be taken up by our flesh and blood and bone. Its beauty, its vibrancy, its life force will become ours.

Food is seductive. If it's there, we eat it. We're still cavemen. That's how they survived. We just have to educate ourselves about who we are and how we function today. We can eat almost anything and still be fine for the moment, but over time we will pay a price. We have to accept that and learn how to act on this knowledge.

Having said all that, I am against dictating to people what they ought to eat. I know what I love, but that's what works for me, my body, and my life. We each have to find things we truly love if we're going to eat them every day for the rest of our lives. Not just chew them and swallow, as if they were medicine—I mean devour them with passion. Be excited by them. Ninety percent of diets fail because the dieters don't love what they're eating. Before long, they revert to their beloved old patterns and put the unhealthy weight right back on, plus a little more.

We can eat badly only thanks to that handy disconnect we've discussed elsewhere in this book: the universal human talent for pretending we don't know what we know. Now, I recognize that some people may need to consult experts when it comes to choosing what to eat and what to avoid. If you're not entirely healthy, you may require a physician or nutritionist to help determine your optimal eating regimen. But most of us don't really need professional advice.

People ask me all the time, "Hey, what should I eat?" and I always answer, "Well, what *should* you eat?" Most folks know the answer as well as I do. And they know it not from the marketing campaigns or fad concepts of the food industry, but from their own natural, intuitive, instinctive sense that fresh, whole foods are the way to go. But if we acknowledge that, then we have to do something about it. And we're not always ready to take that step. So we play the mind game of hiding something from ourselves. Seems to work pretty well. It's a mental device we can't live without.

But all devices get old and wear out at some point, don't they?

When that happens—when we can no longer pretend that our eating habits aren't putting us at definite risk for disease, infirmity, and early death—we're ready to make a change.

All the ex-smokers I know say they loved—*loved*—cigarettes. And yet they all quit. The cultural attitude toward smoking today makes quitting easier than it would have been fifty years ago. We made a big shift where smoking's concerned. It didn't happen overnight. It didn't happen all on its own.

The government began taking steps. It required those scary Surgeon General warnings about cancer and death on the pack. It banned TV advertising. It banished smoking from public places. Before long, it seemed as though the whole world had turned against cigarettes.

Once that happened, it became a lot easier to kick the habit. Nicotine was still as addictive as ever, but once the tide turned, it all went downhill for smoking pretty fast. Not only did people quit, but not as many people started.

What if that happened to bad food, too? All of it—fast food, processed foods, sugar, cheap carbs, unhealthy fats, chemical additives, anything that's making us ill and shortening our lives, the way smoking did. Maybe the government will take the lead again. It has had some success eliminating trans fats and improving labeling. But there are many powerful economic and political interests on the side of harmful food. How do you think all that poison got on our supermarket shelves in the first place?

What would happen if we stopped spending money with corporations that profit from damaging our health and causing our premature death?

Instead of waiting for somebody else to make a change, what if we decide to do it *now*? And what if we took better care of our children and refused to give them unhealthy foods?

We need to question everything when it comes to what we eat. Just because everybody's been eating something forever doesn't make it good for us. Some foods just become part of our culture and so we trust them implicitly, not seeing that they are harming us.

Look at Kellogg's Frosted Flakes, a staple of American breakfast tables for a long, long time. John Harvey Kellogg was a physician who formulated cereals as part of a vegetarian lifestyle. He believed that unhealthy bacteria and microbes in our gut produce toxins during the digestion of proteins, which he said caused a poisoning in the blood. He advocated his cereals as an alternative to animal proteins.

The company that bears his name today has fallen far from his good intentions. We have it to thank for a huge amount of the sugar, refined, nutrition-free grains, and genetically modified ingredients that afflict us today. His company now makes horrible non-food, even though it is a beloved traditional name on supermarket shelves. This is the kind of thing we need to question for our own good.

We need to arrive at the point where we can honestly say, "I love this food because it tastes so good, and it tastes so good because nature made it that way, and nature made it that way because nature and my body are the same thing." Or something like that. Pick your own mantra. Look in the mirror and find something that works.

Just remind yourself: heart disease, cancer, stroke, hypertension, kidney and liver disease, osteoporosis, depression, dementia, adult-onset diabetes—all caused by eating the wrong things. It's not complicated. The choice you make right now creates the next moment you will inhabit.

We all know the practical purpose of eating—to provide us with proper nutrition. What does that mean? The right combination of fats, carbs, and proteins. The necessary vitamins and minerals and fiber. Foods that keep us alkaline. Foods that support our detox systems. Antioxidants to neutralize killer free radicals. Most of the time a food that is good for one of the life forces is good for all of them. This is due to the interconnectedness that binds the life forces together.

The other purpose of eating—just as important as the first one—is to bring us joy and pleasure and satisfaction and to fulfill our bodily desires. To give us three good reasons a day to sit down with people we love, to stop, take a beat, breathe, and give thanks.

It's possible for healthy food to fulfill all its functions. I believe the greatest, best-tasting, and most nutritious food is created exclusively by our planet and not by man. I do not deprive myself of eating's pleasures. Eating when you are aligned on all levels, where your food is nurturing your body and mind and is in synergy with life itself, is one of the greatest pleasures. It just does not come in a package. It never will. Don't take my word for it . . . try it! And let me know how it turns out!

To eat right, there's a long list of foods we can enjoy, and a very short list of things to avoid. So here's what I've done to start you off with some good eating advice: I've made some lists.

As you will see, in my lists I've organized healthy foods into categories, like things that provide protein, or minerals, or fiber, or enzymes, or antioxidants. There are many lists here.

Instead of traditional meal plans, I'm giving you a do-it-yourself kit. Using the lists, I've come up with recipes for thirty sample meals—breakfasts, lunches, and dinners. Each one is satisfying, balanced, tasty, and healthy, if I do say so myself. But feel free to improve on them.

Once you see how I've used the lists to assemble the meals, you'll begin to do it on your own. It's not tricky. It's intuitive. You know what you like to eat. You just need to work that kitchen muscle again!

It would be impossible to list every good food and ingredient on the planet, so don't be constrained by what you find here. Remember, one of the first principles is to get as varied a diet as you can. Each plant food has its own profile of nutrients as well as natural toxins, which is a good reason for not eating too much of any one thing. Seek out variety. We need to paint from as big a palette as possible.

Another good rule is to eat something raw with every meal. I try to be around 70/30—70 percent raw to 30 percent cooked. (Obviously, I'm a big fan of salads and smoothies!) Also, 70 percent veggies and 30 percent all other foods, like fruit, seeds, nuts, whole grains, beans, or tubers. This isn't a hard and fast rule; it's just a good target until it becomes intuitive and natural. Remember, cooking makes foods acidifying, and uncooked ingredients balance out the acidification with an alkalizing influence. Also, cooking kills the natural enzymes, along with some of the phytonutrients and antioxidants, that food contains. Most raw fruits and vegetables contain their own enzymes, which lighten our digestive stress. Raw food also helps our cells stay hydrated. And it just tastes great—a fresh raw fruit or vegetable is totally in-your-face delicious.

But also keep in mind that cooking improves some foods—the heat releases nutrients that we would otherwise miss out on, like the lycopene produced when tomatoes are cooked. And roasting, steaming, boiling, and sautéing also make things taste great. So don't demonize cooking!

Look the lists over and see which foods you like. Some of these you may never have tried. Some you may never have heard of. Give them a chance. Some you may have eaten before and disliked. Give them another chance. Maybe your taste buds have gotten wiser. If you still hate them, move on.

Then assemble your own meals. This is how I eat, except that by now the lists are all in my head. I know the foods I love. I know the things my body needs. I know how to balance my daily eating for optimal results. Listening and being willing to try new things take practice. The best feedback we get is from our own body.

For instance, I know I need to get protein. But I don't worry about getting some in every meal. I know it will add up just from the varied foods I eat throughout the week. I don't get it from meat, fish, or eggs. Instead, it comes from things like beans, kale, chickpeas, or sprouted almonds. I'll prepare a little quinoa, which is a pseudo-grain—a seed, really—and sprinkle it on my salad. These sources don't provide the big wallop of protein you get eating animal flesh. But a little protein from a lot of sources adds up to perfect amino acid profiles with, dare I say, greater biological compatibility, without all the bad stuff that comes along with animal products.

Because a food's color is determined by the phytonutrients it contains, I go for the rainbow—different colors in one sitting. We all need to take care of our immune systems and our ability to detoxify the poisons we take in. So I make sure to eat something that's good for my liver and kidneys.

That's the routine. Try not to overthink it or obsess. Eating is supposed to be fun. I really look forward to mealtimes—we all should. Don't stress over your choices. If you don't eat it today, you'll get it tomorrow or the day after. Try and dazzle yourself with the tasty yet healthy dishes you come up with. If you can manage that, you can't go wrong.

# Kitchen Purge and Re-Stock

**B**efore you begin, do a quick grocery cleanout, followed by a trip to get some necessary staples for your pantry.

## Items to Toss

- White refined sugar (anything containing it, too)
- Homogenized, pasteurized nonorganic milk, yogurt, or butter
- Margarine
- Ordinary table salt
- Refined white flour and anything made from it (breads, tortillas, crackers, pasta, cereal, and so on)
- Deep-fried anything (nuts, etc.)
- Polyunsaturated refined oils (sunflower, corn, soy, canola, and so on)
- Meat and poultry raised by factory farming methods—meaning, most supermarket meat and packaged or cured meat of all kinds
- Eggs from factory farms
- Synthetic beverages (Coke, Pepsi, Kool-Aid, Tang, SunnyD)
- Instant or microwave oatmeal
- All processed microwaved foods (popcorn, instant meals, and so on). And get rid of your microwave, too!
- Non-organic corn (non-GMO)
- Soy sauce
- Boxed processed foods, mixes (cereals, rices, instant packaged meals)
- Plastic storage containers and bags
- Chemical cleaners
- Anything containing high-fructose corn syrup

- Drinks containing sodium benzoate or potassium benzoate
- Foods with butylated hydroxyanisole (BHA), a preservative
- Sodium nitrates and sodium nitrites (processed luncheon meats)
- Blue, green, red, and yellow food coloring (the artificial colors blue 1 and 2, green 3, red 3, and yellow 6 have been linked to thyroid, adrenal, bladder, kidney, and brain cancers)
- Monosodium glutamate (MSG)

Now that you've cleared out some space, here are a few staples to buy. Get organic and/or wild-harvested products when possible:

# Pantry Staples

- Herbal teas
- Fermented beverages such as kefir and kombucha
- Nut milks, including almond and coconut
- Nut butters, including almond and cashew
- Natural salts such as Celtic sea salt, and Himalayan salt
- Spices—cinnamon, clove, cardamom, allspice, turmeric, and so on
- Fermented products such as kimchi, sauerkraut, and miso
- Garbanzo miso paste
- Apple cider vinegar
- Sweeteners such as stevia, coconut palm sugar, yacon syrup, molasses, agave, and raw honey
- Amino products like Coconut Secret Aminos and Bragg's Liquid Aminos
- Steel-cut oats
- Cold-pressed, organic extra-virgin olive oil, coconut oil, grape-seed oil, sacha inchi oil, avocado oil, and toasted sesame oil
- Raw organic nuts and seeds, soaked and sprouted whenever possible
- Ezekiel sprouted bread
- Ezekiel sprouted-corn tortillas
- Organic local fresh herbs, veggies, and fruits
- Organic sprouts

- Organic free-range/pasture-raised meat, if you're eating meat
- Unpasteurized, organic grass-fed milk and butter and organic free-range eggs
- Glass storage containers and bottles

## Some kitchen appliances you may want:

- Vitamix (high-powered blender for smoothies, soups, purees, and so on)
- Dehydrator (low-temperature cooking for preservation of nutrients and enzymes; a great kitchen tool for making snacks such as kale chips and dried fruits and veggies)
- Toaster oven (for conserving energy; faster than a bigger oven)
- Steamer (keeps the veggies out of water and in the steam, minimizing nutrient loss)
- Coffee grinder (for grinding dried spices and seeds)

# Water Maker Options

- Countertop distiller (in a glass bottle, with added crystal salt for drinking)
- Air-to-water machine (takes water out of the air and filters it for drinking)
- Reverse osmosis filters (OK if you add Himalayan crystal salt in a glass bottle)
- Vortex machine (stirs and structures water)

# The Foods We'll Eat and Why

## Protein

You'll notice I don't recommend any animal sources, except for the occasional organic free-range egg. As I've said elsewhere in this book, if you do eat meat, make it organic and humanely raised on pasture or (for chicken) free-range. And don't overdo it.

- Almonds
- Beans, any variety
- Chickpeas or hummus
- Eggs—whole, organic, and free-range, yolks as lightly cooked as possible—even raw—because high heat kills off the nutrients
- Kale
- Lentils
- Pumpkin seeds
- Quinoa
- Seaweed—nori, kombu, sea lettuce
- Sunflower seeds
- Tempeh, organic three-grain

## Good Fats

Fats are healthy, as long as we get the right ones. The body doesn't produce essential fatty acids, so we need to get them from what we eat and through proper supplementation (see "How to Supplement"). Remember, fats exist not just in oils but in vegetables and nuts, which may be the healthiest source of all.

- Almonds and almond butter
- Avocados
- Chia seed, freshly ground
- Coconut oil
- Cold-pressed extra-virgin olive oil
- Cold-pressed organic flax oil
- Freshly ground flaxseed
- Raw milk or butter, unpasteurized, from organic grass-fed goats or cows
- Sacha inchi oil
- Walnuts

# Minerals

Even though these are nonliving substances, it's best to get them from living foods. We require them to keep us alive and healthy. Around 4 percent of our total body mass is made up of minerals, mostly calcium, potassium, magnesium, phosphorus, sodium, and sulfur.

- Alfalfa sprouts
- Broccoli
- Cabbage
- Garlic
- Hazelnuts
- Kale
- Natural unrefined salts like Himalayan salt or Celtic sea salt
- Oats
- Seaweed—wakame, nori, or kelp
- Sunflower seeds

## Calcium
Contributes to bones and teeth but also serves pivotal roles in neurotransmitter, cell communication, muscle (including heart), and fertility functions. It's the main buffering backup system when the body is in acidosis.

- Apricots
- Brussels sprouts

- Butternut squash
- Cabbages
- Chard
- Dandelion leaves
- Figs
- Kelp
- Pistachios
- Plums
- Sesame seeds or tahini
- Spinach
- Turnips

## Magnesium

Found in every human cell; pivotal in ATP biological activity and DNA/RNA synthesis. Responsible for nutrient uptake of the cells as well as helping facilitate fat metabolism and hormone and insulin regulation.

- Asparagus
- Avocado
- Bananas
- Beet greens
- Brazil nuts
- Brown rice (use sparingly)
- Cashews
- Kiwis
- Peas
- Prunes
- Squash

## Potassium

Essential to all cellular functions, responsible for communication between nerve and muscle cells. Needed for fluid and electrolyte balance, which directly influence blood pressure and pH control.

- Acorn squash
- Broccoli
- Cabbage
- Carrots

- Cherries
- Currant
- Kiwi fruit
- Mushrooms (white)
- Peanuts
- Sweet potato

## Iron

Mineral required for vital biological functions such as oxygen transport in the blood and ATP creation in the mitochondria. It forms part of the enzymes required for antioxidant functions and many other actions within the body.

- Coconuts
- Legumes (beans and peas)
- Macadamia nuts
- Oats (traditional steel-cut)
- Quinoa
- Raisins
- Sesame seeds
- Sun-dried tomatoes
- Swiss chard
- Watercress

## Copper

Copper helps to regulate cholesterol (the essential steroid hormone and cell membrane building block) and glucose metabolism, fights infection, helps tissue repair, and neutralizes free-radical scavenging.

- Apricots
- Cashews
- Coconut
- Hazelnuts
- Kale
- Peaches
- Pecans
- Portobello mushrooms

- Shiitake mushrooms
- Walnuts

## Zinc

Key trace element with biological roles from metabolism of RNA and DNA to reproductive organ growth. It forms the structural and bioactive part of over a hundred important enzymes.

- Asparagus
- Green peas
- Lemongrass
- Napa cabbage
- Oats
- Pecans
- Prunes
- Pumpkin seeds
- Shiitake mushrooms
- Spinach

## Phosphorus

Nature provides phosphorus in a wide range of foods. The basic structure of DNA/RNA is made up of phosphorus, and cell membranes also contain it as a main structural component. It turns enzyme activity on or off, helps to strengthen bones, and has many other functions in our bodies.

- Alfalfa sprouts
- Avocados
- Broccoli
- Celery
- Chia seeds
- Kiwi fruit
- Pistachios
- Watercress
- Wild rice
- Zucchini

## *Manganese*

Essential trace nutrient that's bonded as a cofactor to a multitude of active enzymes, assisting in many bodily functions. Essential antioxidants depend on this mineral for proper liver, brain, and bone health.

- Blueberries
- Chilies (any color)
- Collard greens
- Currant
- Eggplant
- Garlic
- Grapes
- Leeks
- Pumpkin seeds
- Raspberries

## *Selenium*

Essential for the heart, blood, brain, and thyroid. Evidence shows that it also increases the action of antioxidants.

- Asparagus
- Brazil nuts
- Broccoli
- Brussels sprouts
- Coconut
- Garlic
- Grapefruit
- Mushrooms (shiitake, portobello)
- Spinach
- Sunflower seeds

# Vitamins

## *Vitamin A*

Essential fat-soluble vitamin indispensable for proper vision, skin, antioxidant function, and immune system maintenance.

- Avocado
- Bell peppers
- Cantaloupe
- Carrots
- Chili peppers (especially the orange, red, and yellow ones; the brighter the color, the more beta carotene)
- Cod-liver oil
- Collard greens
- Mangoes
- Organic grass-fed butter
- Organic free-range eggs, yolks still liquid, or even raw
- Spinach
- Sweet potatoes

## *Vitamin B*

A group of eight chemically different water-soluble vitamins, found throughout the plant and animal kingdoms. They play key roles in healthy cell function and biological functions. The B vitamin group has almost limitless benefits for the functioning of optimal health.

- Brown rice (use sparingly)
- Cabbage
- Fermented foods such as kimchi, sauerkraut, some homemade pickles, and traditional yogurt
- Legumes
- Nutritional yeast
- Nuts—almonds, Brazil nuts, cashews
- Peanuts

- Quinoa
- Seeds—chia, sunflower seeds, and so on
- Wild mushrooms

## Vitamin C

Water-soluble essential nutrient found primarily but not exclusively in citric fruits. Responsible for key enzymatic reactions involved in collagen formation and has a wide range of active roles in maintaining human functions—immune, antihistamine, antioxidant, and capillary, among others.

- Bok choy (Chinese cabbage)
- Broccoli
- Brussels sprouts
- Citrus fruits (mandarin, orange, lemon, and so on)
- Kiwi fruit
- Papaya
- Peppers (bell and chili peppers)
- Pineapple
- Raspberries
- Strawberries

## Vitamin D

Vitamin D is primarily synthesized from the cholesterol in skin exposed to sunlight. Vital for key biological functions such as calcium and phosphate gut uptake, bone and neuromuscular health, immune health, and many other important roles. The number-one nutrient for the regulation of all cancers.

- Certain mushrooms, including chanterelle, oyster, portobello, shiitake, and cremini (better if exposed to UVA/UVB)

## *Vitamin E*

Responsible for antioxidant activity, tissue repair, neurological functions, and much more.

- Almonds
- Avocados
- Brazil nuts
- Chia
- Cod-liver oil
- Cold-pressed extra-virgin olive oil
- Freshly ground flaxseed
- Peanut butter
- Quinoa
- Sunflower seeds
- Walnuts

## *Vitamin K*

Predominately activated by gut bacteria. Important for blood clotting and bone and cardiovascular health.

- Basil
- Beet greens
- Bok choy (Chinese cabbage)
- Broccoli
- Brussels sprouts
- Kale
- Pumpkin seeds
- Spinach
- Turnips

# Alkalizing Foods

- Alliums—onion, garlic, chives, shallot, leek
- Almonds
- Apple cider vinegar
- Berries
- Chili peppers
- Citrus (fresh)

- Cruciferous vegetables—broccoli, cabbage, cauliflower
- Cucurbits—cucumber, watermelon, squash, pumpkin, cantaloupe
- Greens—kale, red-leaf lettuce, romaine, mint, parsley
- Herbs—sage, oregano, basil, and so on
- Himalayan salt
- Seaweed
- Spices—ginger, cinnamon, mustard, turmeric, curry
- Sprouts
- Stevia

# Fiber

Some fiber assists our digestive tract to do its jobs properly. Other forms of it are consumed by microbes and fermented into bioactive compounds. All are necessary.

- All whole veggies and fruits
- Apples
- Beans
- Chia seeds
- Chickpeas
- Coconut (whole)
- Freshly ground flaxseed
- Oats
- Pumpkin seeds
- Quinoa
- Walnut

# Detoxifying Foods

The human body has evolved and adapted with very effective mechanisms to eliminate toxins, waste, and metabolic debris. Certain foods contain compounds and elements that greatly assist these mechanisms.

- All fruits and vegetables
- Berries such as cranberries, blueberries, and blackberries

- Chilies
- Fermented foods such as kimchi, sauerkraut, and kefir
- Garlic
- Greens such as collard, mustard, dandelion, and beet
- Herbs such as oregano, cilantro, basil, mint, and parsley
- Raw apple cider vinegar
- Seaweed
- Sprouts
- Turmeric

# Antioxidants

Foods that counteract the harmful oxidation caused by free radicals.

- Artichoke hearts
- Avocado
- Beans
- Berries such as blueberries and raspberries
- Cranberries
- Oregano
- Pecans
- Pomegranates
- Prunes
- Quinoa
- Spices such as cloves, cumin, cinnamon, curry, turmeric, and vanilla

# Anti-Inflammatory Foods

Stress and dehydration create chronic inflammation that can lead to chronic diseases. These foods assist the body in regulating inflammation and nourishing the damaged areas.

- Alliums such as onion, garlic, and leeks
- Cold-pressed extra-virgin olive oil
- Fermented foods such as traditional yogurt and kefir

- Freshly ground flaxseed
- Ginger
- Green tea
- Hazelnuts
- Macadamia nuts
- Rosemary
- Seaweed—kombu, nori, kelp
- Turmeric

# Prebiotics

Foods that create favorable conditions for the healthy microbes our bodies need.

- Agave
- Alliums such as leeks, onion, and garlic
- Apples
- Asparagus
- Bananas
- Cruciferous vegetables such as cabbage, broccoli, and kale
- Greens such as dandelion, beet, mustard, amaranth, and collard
- Oats
- Papaya
- Quinoa
- Walnuts

# Probiotics

Fermentation is an ancient process that gives food a longer shelf life but also introduces beneficial flora into the intestines, where we need them.

- Apple cider vinegar
- Fermented foods such as sauerkraut
- Kimchi

- Kombucha
- Miso
- Olives
- Plain traditional kefir
- Plain traditional yogurt
- Raw or low-temp-processed cacao
- Tempeh

# Immune System Support

Certain foods supply us with essential nutrients and important nonessential molecules that play important roles in activating and regulating our body's defense system.

- Aloe vera
- Echinacea
- Garlic
- Ginger
- Goldenseal
- Mushrooms—shiitake and turkey tail
- Onion
- Organic raw local honey
- Oxygen and alkaline foods (see page 219)

# Good for Your Brain

This organ is the most metabolically active part of your body, and debatably the most important, too. (At least in its own opinion.) It requires lots of nutrients for proper function.

- Blueberries
- Brazil nuts
- Coconut oil
- Cod-liver oil
- Green tea
- Nuts such as hazelnut, macadamia, pecan, and walnut
- Quinoa
- Rosemary

# Good for Your Blood

Foods help to make new blood but also support the organs responsible for filtering and cleansing it.

- Alliums such as leeks, garlic, and onion
- Beets
- Chia seeds
- Chili peppers
- Cilantro
- Citrus
- Coconut water
- Cold-pressed organic juice from cereal grasses like wheat, barley, and kamut
- Parsley
- Pomegranates
- Seaweed—nori, kelp, wakame

# Stress

The brain and the adrenals in particular help us to cope with stress, so we need to eat foods that support those organs in their work.

- Chamomile
- Ginseng
- Licorice root
- Passionflower
- Raw nuts and seeds such as almonds, pecans, Brazil nuts, and sunflower seeds
- Schizandra berries
- Scullcap
- St.-John's-wort
- Valerian

# Energy

Boosting your body with a spark, a feeling of balance and vigor.

- Apple cider vinegar
- Chili peppers
- Ginseng
- Green tea
- Kimchi
- Raw local honey
- Quinoa
- Reishi mushrooms
- Sprouts—bean, broccoli, alfalfa
- Yerba mate

# Joints

Foods can support things like cartilage, synovial fluid, collagen, and other joint-related structures, and also reduce inflammation and increase blood flow.

- Avocado
- Black pepper
- Chili peppers
- Coconut oil
- Cod-liver oil
- Cold-pressed extra-virgin olive oil
- Ginger
- Nuts (best if soaked or sprouted)
- Pineapple
- Turmeric

# Sex

When the body is unhealthy, the desire for sex is diminished. Phytonutrients have been proven in the lab to support libido.

- Avocado
- Cacao
- Fenugreek seeds
- Garlic
- Ginseng
- Pumpkin seeds
- Quinoa
- Raw local honey
- Vanilla

# Skin

Local disturbances as well as internal ones are quickly manifested in our skin, and the foods we eat have a metabolic impact on our surfaces.

- Almonds
- Avocado
- Berries such as blueberries and strawberries
- Brazil nuts
- Citrus fruit
- Coconut oil
- Cod-liver oil
- Pumpkin seeds
- Quinoa
- Sesame oil

# Eyes

Foods that provide phytonutrients protect our eyes and the nerves around them.

- Avocado
- Bilberries
- Blueberries
- Eyebright
- Fennel
- Grape seeds
- Greens such as kale, dandelion, and romaine
- Green tea
- Milk thistle
- Saffron
- Tomatoes

# Muscles

Bone and joint health depend on the health of our skeletal muscles, and metabolism related to body mass is in great part directly correlated to muscle health.

- Almonds
- Brazil nuts
- Chia seeds
- Eggs (organic free-range )
- Garlic
- Leafy greens (kale, spinach)
- Pecans
- Pine pollen
- Pumpkin seeds
- Quinoa
- Walnuts

# Ten Great Crucifers

Cruciferous vegetables are known to possess high amounts of fiber and vitamin C. Many phytonutrients are found only in crucifers.

- Arugula
- Bok choy
- Broccoli
- Brussels sprouts
- Cabbage
- Cauliflower
- Collard greens
- Kale
- Mustard greens
- Watercress

# Great Berries

Nourishing, protecting, balancing, and detoxifying; new research is constantly providing us with further evidence of berries' goodness. Plus, they're delicious.

- Açai berries
- Blackberries
- Blueberries
- Cranberries
- Goji berries
- Goldenberries (Incan berries)
- Mulberries
- Raspberries
- Strawberries

# Ten Great Nuts

The outdated view is that they're fattening. Now we know they provide necessary healthy fats and other nutrients that aid the cardiovascular system, metabolism, even weight management. People who eat nuts daily live longer than those who don't. Eat them raw, sprouted, or soaked whenever possible.

- Almonds
- Brazil nuts
- Cashews
- Coconut
- Hazelnuts
- Macadamia nuts
- Pecans
- Pine nuts
- Pistachios
- Walnuts

# Ten Great Legumes

These nutrient-dense foods can be prepared in many ways—sprouted, fermented, dried, roasted, boiled—and benefit digestive, cardiac, nervous, hepatic, and cellular health. Some people fear beans because they sometimes make us fart. Grow up!

- Black beans
- Chickpeas
- Fava beans
- Kidney beans
- Lentils
- Mung beans
- Navy beans
- Peanuts
- Peas
- Soybeans (organic, non-GMO)

# Ten Great Seeds

Seeds are nature's nutritional warehouse, containing all the basic elements to nourish and maintain a properly functioning body. They're extremely rich in minerals, vitamins, and plant compounds.

- Apple seeds
- Cacao (raw chocolate is actually a seed)
- Chia seeds (soaked or freshly ground)
- Freshly ground flaxseed
- Oats
- Pomegranate seeds
- Pumpkin seeds
- Quinoa
- Sesame seeds
- Sunflower seeds

# Ten Great Leafy Green Vegetables

The most abundant color in nature is green, so it is no surprise that some of nature's most nutrient-dense foods are green as well. Highly available, inexpensive, and easy to prepare, they transform the energy of the sun, combining it with oxygen, water, and minerals to help us with detoxifying, nourishing, fortifying, and prevention.

- Arugula
- Bok choy
- Cilantro
- Collards
- Dandelion greens
- Kale
- Lettuce
- Mustard greens

- Spinach
- Watercress

# Great Anti-Cancer Foods

- Alliums such as garlic, onion, and chives
- All leafy greens (kale, spinach, etc.)
- Beans—black, green, kidney, and mung, among others
- Berries
- Cereal grasses—wheat, barley, and so on
- Fermented foods such as yogurt, kefir, and kimchi
- Nuts—almond, Brazil, and so on
- Quinoa
- Spices such as curry, turmeric, and ginger
- Sweet potatoes
- Tea—green and rooibos

# Ten Great Heart Foods

- Avocado
- Berries
- Carrots
- Fatty fish such as sardines, herring, and anchovies
- Freshly ground flaxseed
- Legumes
- Nuts
- Oatmeal
- Olive oil
- Spinach

# Anti-High Blood Pressure Foods

- Apples
- Bell peppers
- Cabbage
- Celery juice, warmed
- Garlic

- Greens
- Kiwi fruit
- Spinach
- Strawberries
- Sweet potatoes
- Tempeh
- Tomatoes, raw
- Watermelon

# Anti-Heartburn Foods

- Aloe vera
- Apple cider vinegar
- Asian pears
- Bananas
- Brown rice
- Celery and celery juice
- Ginger root
- Pineapple
- Water

# Great Color Foods

Hue is a reliable indicator of high-nutrient, high-polyphenol, and high-antioxidant content. We need to get some of every shade. Eat your colors!

## *Reds*

- Beets
- Bell peppers
- Cherries
- Chili peppers
- Cranberries
- Pomegranates
- Raspberries

- Red apples
- Red beans
- Strawberries
- Tomatoes
- Watermelon

## Oranges

- Apricots
- Bell peppers
- Cantaloupes
- Carrots
- Citrus—oranges, tangerines
- Eggs—organic and free-range, yolks uncooked
- Mangoes
- Nectarines
- Papayas
- Peaches
- Pumpkins
- Squash
- Sweet potatoes
- Yams

## Yellows

- Bananas
- Butter—organic and grass-fed
- Chickpeas
- Corn
- Grapefruit
- Lemons
- Peaches
- Pineapples
- Potatoes
- Rutabagas/turnips
- Spices such as saffron, curcumin, turmeric, and ginger
- Squash

*Blues and Purples*

- Blackberries
- Black currants
- Blue corn
- Blue potatoes
- Blueberries
- Eggplant
- Figs
- Grapes
- Plums
- Purple cabbages
- Purple yams
- Radicchio
- Shallots (purple ones)
- Turnips

# Ten Great Common Spices

Spices were the first superfoods, and even today in some parts of the world they hold sacred status. They can be antibiotic, antimicrobial, antifungal, anti-inflammatory, antioxidant, and restorative, and many more benefits are constantly being discovered.

- Cardamom
- Chili powder
- Cinnamon
- Clove
- Curry
- Garlic
- Ginger
- Mustard
- Natural salt such as Himalayan or Celtic sea salt
- Turmeric

# Great Common Herbs

Herbs are nature's medicine, proven through millennia of traditional use across the globe to support, detoxify, tone, and nourish specific organs, tissues, and systems.

- Basil
- Chamomile
- Cilantro
- Dill
- Mint
- Oregano
- Rosemary
- Sage
- Tarragon

# Healthy Sweeteners

The craving for sweetness is hardwired in our genes, further exploited by the food industry. But there are healthy alternatives to sugar and high-fructose corn syrup.

- Agave syrup, raw organic, preferably from *Agave salmiana*
- Blackstrap molasses
- Coconut sugar
- Date sugar
- Honey, raw organic and local
- Lo han guo
- Maple syrup, grade B, traditionally tapped and processed
- Stevia
- Yacon syrup

# Healthy Drinks (Aside from Water)

- Coconut milk and water
- Fruit juices/smoothies, freshly juiced from whole fruit
- Green tea

- Green veggie juices, freshly juiced
- Herbal tea
- Kefir, made with water or whole organic raw milk
- Kombucha
- Nut and seed milks such as oat, almond, and hemp

# Some Nutrient-Dense Superfoods

There are many, but I like these best.

- Acai
- Acerola
- Algae—blue green, chlorella, spirulina
- Aloe
- Amla
- Ashwagandha
- Astragalus
- Baobab
- Cacao
- Camu camu
- Goji
- Golden berries (Incan berries)
- Maca
- Moringa
- Mushrooms—chaga, reishi, maitake, cordyceps
- Rhodiola
- Sacha inchi
- Tonkat ali

# Darin's Ten-Day Eating Plan

Three meals a day plus a snack, just to get you started. Once you're in the habit of eating this way, you'll be able to come up with your own menus and recipes.

DAY 1
BREAKFAST: Power Quinoa Porridge
LUNCH: Rainbow Salad
SNACK: Power Trail Mix
DINNER: Kale, Seeds, Tomato, and Tempeh

DAY 2
BREAKFAST: Berry Good Morning
LUNCH: Protein Power Kale Salad
SNACK: Almond-Date Balls
DINNER: Tempeh Tacos

DAY 3
BREAKFAST: Begin the Day with Greatness Green Smoothie
LUNCH: Quinoa Salad with Herbs and Nuts
SNACK: Brain Turn-On Nut Medley
DINNER: Mushroom Ceviche with Wild Green Salad

DAY 4
BREAKFAST: "Rise" Steel-Cut Oat Breakfast
LUNCH: Whatever's Left in the Fridge Salad
SNACK: Hulk Snack
DINNER: Mung Bean Burrito

DAY 5

BREAKFAST: Shakeology Double Chocolate Power Vegan
Smoothie
LUNCH: Kale and Seaweed Salad
SNACK: Easy Peel-and-Dip
DINNER: Simple "Cheezy" Quinoa and Broccoli

DAY 6

BREAKFAST: Seasonal Fruit Bowl
LUNCH: "A Great Marriage" Quinoa and Kale
SNACK: Creamy Afternoon Pick-Me-Up Smoothie
DINNER: Split Pea Soup

DAY 7

BREAKFAST: What a Blast Morning Smoothie
LUNCH: Hummus Wrap
SNACK: Homemade Guaco-Love
DINNER: Lentil Salad

DAY 8

BREAKFAST: Back to Life Fresh Smoothie
LUNCH: Tempeh Salad
SNACK: Almond Butter Heaven
DINNER: Sweet Potato Soup

DAY 9

BREAKFAST: Morning Pudding
LUNCH: Raw Lettuce Wraps
SNACK: Zinging Avocado Cacao Pudding
DINNER: Wild Rice and Mushrooms

DAY 10

BREAKFAST: Tempeh Breakfast Scramble
LUNCH: Red Quinoa Delight
SNACK: Berry Heaven
DINNER: Darin's Pizza

# Day 1

## Breakfast:

### Power Quinoa Porridge

½ cup sprouted quinoa or steel-cut oats, washed to remove dirt and extra starch and cooked

2 tsp raw cacao nibs

1 tsp raw cacao powder

½ tsp maca powder

½ tsp cinnamon powder

Pinch habanero pepper powder (optional)

½ cup almond milk (see page 267), coconut milk (see page 268), or coconut water

1 tablespoon yacon, agave syrup, or raw honey, or for lower sugar and calories use stevia

Use precooked quinoa, or wash and cook quinoa according to package instructions. Mix all ingredients in a bowl and top with cacao nibs.

*Makes 1 serving*

PER SERVING: 288 CALORIES, 5 G FAT, 52 G CARBS, 8 G PROTEIN

## Lunch:

### Rainbow Salad

1 cup romaine lettuce

1 cup kale

1 cup red-leaf lettuce

½ cup broccoli

½ cup red pepper

½ cup yellow pepper

1 tbsp kimchi (fermented cabbage)

½ cup cucumber

½ cup heirloom tomato

1 tablespoon sprouted or soaked almonds (see page 267)

## *Dressing:*

2 tbsp toasted sesame oil

1 tsp garbanzo miso paste

2 tbsp Bragg's Liquid Aminos or Coconut Secret Aminos

1 avocado

2 tbsp apple cider vinegar (Bragg's)

Juice from 1 lemon

Combine salad ingredients in a bowl. Add dressing ingredients to a blender and blend on high. Pour dressing over salad and toss.

*Makes 2 servings*

PER SERVING: 447 CALORIES, 32 G FAT, 39 G CARBS, 12 G PROTEIN

## *Snack:*

## Power Trail Mix

½ cup nuts—soaked or sprouted raw cashews, raw almonds, raw walnuts, or a combination

2 tbsp goji berries or dried cranberries

2 tbsp cacao nibs

2 tbsp golden berries or cut-up date chunks

½ tsp Himalayan salt

Mix in a bowl. Store extra for future snacks.

*Makes four ¼ cup servings*

PER SERVING: 198 CALORIES, 12 G FAT, 19 G CARBS, 6 G PROTEIN

## Dinner:

### Kale, Seeds, Tomato, and Tempeh

1 loaf organic three-grain tempeh, cut in strips

Sesame or coconut oil for sautéing

8–10 large kale leaves, chopped

½ cup romaine lettuce, chopped

8 plum or 1 medium heirloom tomato, chopped

½ cup red onion, chopped

1 cup fresh basil, roughly chopped

½ cup fresh cilantro, roughly chopped

2 tbsp walnuts

½ cup chopped apple

½ cup sesame or avocado oil

½ tsp Himalayan salt

Mixed dried herbs, to taste

Season the tempeh with salt and sauté in a little sesame oil or coconut oil, 3–5 minutes on each side. Cut the tempeh strips in half.

Combine kale, romaine lettuce, tomato, red onion, basil, cilantro, apples, and walnuts in a medium bowl. Add oil, Himalayan salt, and mixed herbs. Toss salad, and top with tempeh.

*Makes 2 servings*

PER SERVING: 693 CALORIES, 48 G FAT, 46 G CARBS, 29 G PROTEIN

TOTAL DAILY VALUES: 1,625 CALORIES, 97 G FAT, 155 G CARBS, 53 G PROTEIN

# Day 2

## Breakfast:

### Berry Good Morning

2 cups seasonal mixed berries (cranberries, strawberries,
blueberries, raspberries, etc.)

½ cup coconut shavings

DRESSING:

½ cup coconut water

2 tbsp fresh mint leaves, chopped

2 tbsp cashew butter or coconut butter (coconut water blended
with coconut meat)

½ medium avocado

Wash berries and place in a bowl. Use a blender to mix sauce
ingredients together, and pour on top of berries. Sprinkle
with coconut shavings.

*Makes 1 serving*

PER SERVING: 451 CALORIES, 27 G FAT, 49 G CARBS, 11 G PROTEIN

## Lunch:

### Protein Power Kale Salad

2 cups chopped kale

5 kalamata olives

1 green onion, chopped

½ cup jicama, chopped

½ cup mixed green and red bell peppers

½ avocado, sliced

2 tbsp pine nuts

DRESSING:

⅓ cup lemon juice

⅓ cup sesame or avocado oil

1 tbsp onion powder

½ cup water

½ tsp garlic powder

Mixed dried herbs, to taste

All-purpose seasoning (unsalted)

1 tsp Himalayan salt

Combine salad ingredients in bowl. Blend dressing ingredients until smooth and creamy. Add 2 tbsp dressing to salad, and toss.

*Makes 1 serving*

PER SERVING: 288 CALORIES, 18 G FAT, 37 G CARBS, 6 G PROTEIN

## *Snack:*

## Almond-Date Balls

3 Medjool dates, mashed

2 tbsp almond butter

Cinnamon

Mash ingredients together and roll into balls. Dust with cinnamon.

*Makes 2 servings*

PER SERVING: 189 CALORIES, 8 G FAT, 31 G CARBS, 5 G PROTEIN

## Dinner:

### Tempeh Tacos

1 block tempeh, chopped

½ cup each red and green bell pepper, chopped

3 green onions, chopped

2 tbsp red onion, chopped

½ cup chopped yellow squash

¼ cup chopped portabello mushrooms

½ cup chopped green zucchini

Mixed dried herbs, to taste

½ tsp Himalayan salt, or to taste

6 Ezekiel sprouted-corn tortillas

½ cup romaine lettuce, chopped

5 cherry tomatoes, chopped

1 tbsp Bragg's Liquid Aminos or Coconut Secret Aminos, or a dash of Himalayan salt

Sauté tempeh, peppers, onions, squash, portobello mushrooms, and zucchini in a pan with a layer of coconut oil until soft. Season with mixed herbs and salt.

Fill tortilla shells with vegetable mixture and bake for 10 minutes at 300°F in regular oven, or in a dehydrator for 1 hour at 130°F.

Top with lettuce, mushrooms, tomatoes, and aminos or salt.

*Makes two 3-taco servings*

PER SERVING: 478 CALORIES, 14 G FAT, 61 G CARBS, 26 G PROTEIN

TOTAL DAILY VALUES: 1,520 CALORIES, 77 G FAT, 184 G CARBS, 50 G PROTEIN

# Day 3

## *Breakfast:*

### Begin the Day with Greatness Green Smoothie

½ large banana, frozen

½ cup mango, frozen

1 cup fresh spinach (add some kale for an extra kick of protein)

½ cup blueberries

1 cup almond milk (see page 267), coconut milk (see page 268), or coconut water

2 tbsp soaked chia seeds (see page 268)

2 ice cubes

Pinch cinnamon

Put almond milk and ice in blender. Add the rest of the ingredients, and blend until smooth.

*Makes 1 serving*

PER SERVING: 292 CALORIES, 13 G FAT, 43 G CARBS, 8 G PROTEIN

## *Lunch:*

### Quinoa Salad with Herbs and Nuts

2 cups quinoa, cooked

½ cup pecans (or substitute pine nuts or almonds)

½ cup fresh mint, chopped

½ cup fresh parsley, chopped

3 scallions (green onions), chopped

1 tbsp coconut or avocado oil

1 tbsp lemon or lime juice

1 tsp garlic powder

½ tsp Himalayan salt

Black pepper to taste

Use precooked quinoa, or wash and cook quinoa according to package instructions. Combine all ingredients in a bowl, and toss. For an extra hint of sweetness, add goji berries or dried cranberries.

*Makes 2 servings*

PER SERVING: 525 CALORIES, 31 G FAT, 13 G CARBS, 6 G PROTEIN

## Snack:

### Brain Turn-On Nut Medley

10 cashews, soaked
12 soaked or sprouted almonds
5 soaked walnuts
Cranberries and/or chopped dates (optional)

Mix and enjoy.

*Makes 1 serving*

PER SERVING: 363 CALORIES, 31 G FAT, 16 G CARBS, 13 G PROTEIN

## Dinner:

### Mushroom Ceviche with Wild Green Salad

1 cup chopped portobello mushroom (or use local, seasonal varieties—turkey tail, enoki, oyster, white, shiitake, chanterelles, maitake)
Juice of 2-3 large lemons
½ tsp Himalayan salt
1 cup quinoa, cooked
½ cup alfalfa sprouts

SALAD:

2 cups mixed greens—spinach, radicchio, watercress, dandelion, etc.

1 tbsp fresh ginger, shredded

½ tbsp extra-virgin organic olive oil or toasted sesame oil or make your favorite dressing

½ cup carrots, fermented or fresh

½ cup beets, fermented or fresh

½ cup green beans, fermented or fresh

½ tsp Himalayan salt to taste

Mix chopped mushrooms, lemon juice, and Himalayan salt in a bowl. Allow mushrooms to absorb juice.

Cook quinoa according to the package directions. Top with mushrooms, and then with sprouts. Put aside.

Mix all salad ingredients together in a bowl. Serve with ceviche.

*Makes 1 serving*

PER SERVING: 544 CALORIES, 18 G FAT, 84 G CARBS, 42 G PROTEIN

TOTAL DAILY VALUES: 1,724 CALORIES, 92 G FAT, 196 G CARBS, 48 G PROTEIN

# Day 4

## Breakfast:

### "Rise" Steel-Cut Oat Breakfast

1 cup steel-cut oats, teff, or fonio

1 cup almond milk (see page 267)

2 tbsp soaked chia seeds (see page 268)

½ tsp cinnamon

½ tsp vanilla extract

1 tbsp agave syrup, honey, yacon syrup, or stevia

2 tbsp almonds, cashews, or pistachios

½ cup berries

½ banana, sliced, if desired

Prepare steel-cut oats, teff, or fonio according to package instructions. Once cereal is prepared, add almond milk, soaked chia seeds, cinnamon, vanilla extract, honey (or sweetener of choice), and mix together. Let cereal cool to room temperature or place in refrigerator.

Once cooled, add nuts, berries, and banana, if using.

*Makes 2 servings*

PER SERVING: 310 CALORIES, 14 G FAT, 42 G CARBS, 9 G PROTEIN

## Lunch:

### Whatever's Left in the Fridge Salad

½ cup spinach

½ cup kale

10 sweet cherry tomatoes, cut in half

½ cup shredded carrot

½ cup romaine lettuce

½ cup jicama, chopped

½ cup each red and yellow bell pepper, chopped

2 tsp walnuts

½ avocado, chopped

½ cup chopped red onion

½ cup chopped cucumber

DRESSING (MAKES ABOUT 1 CUP):

½ cup apple cider vinegar

1 Medjool date, smashed

½ tsp Himalayan salt

½ tsp mixed dried herbs, or to taste

½ cup avocado, coconut, or sesame oil

Mix all salad ingredients in a bowl. Blend dressing ingredients in a blender, or with a hand mixer. Add 2 tbsp of dressing to salad. Save the rest of the dressing in the refrigerator for later, or share!

*Makes 1 serving*

PER SERVING: 358 CALORIES, 21 G FAT, 49 G CARBS, 10 G PROTEIN

## Snack:

## Hulk Snack

½ cup almond butter

1 tbsp spirulina

2 tbsp soaked chia seeds (see page 268)

1 green apple, sliced

¼ tsp cinnamon

Mix together almond butter, spirulina, chia, and cinnamon. Spread half of this mixture on green apple slices. Save the rest for later, or share!

PER SERVING: 363 CALORIES, 21 G FAT, 15 G CARBS, 24 G PROTEIN

*Dinner:*

## Mung Bean Burrito

1 cup mung beans

3 cups water

½ tsp Himalayan salt

6 large Ezekiel sprouted-corn tortillas

1 tbsp hummus or Veganaise

½ cup red, yellow, and/or green peppers, sliced

½ cup yellow squash and/or zucchini, sliced

½ heirloom tomato, sliced

½ cup kale

1 avocado

Bring water to a simmer in pot. Add mung beans and salt and simmer until tender, about 25–30 minutes. Set aside 2 or 3 tbsp, and store the rest for other uses.

Preheat oven to 300°F. Warm tortillas in preheating oven for 1–2 minutes.

Take out tortillas, and spread a thin layer of hummus or Veganaise on each. Add in layers: 2 tbsp mung beans, peppers, squash, tomato, and kale. Fold burrito and tie closed with a piece of tin foil folded into a strip and twisted around burrito to secure contents.

Bake for 20–30 minutes in regular oven at 300°F.

Take out of oven and add sliced avocado.

---

PER SERVING: 376 CALORIES, 16 G FAT, 50 G CARBS, 12 G PROTEIN*

TOTAL DAILY VALUES: 1,407 CALORIES, 71 G FAT, 167 G CARBS, 56 G PROTEIN

*ACCOMPANIED BY A RAW SALAD AT THAT MEAL, OR THAT DAY.

# Day 5

## *Breakfast:*

### Shakeology Double Chocolate Power Vegan Smoothie

1–2 cups coconut water or coconut milk (see page 268)

2–3 ice cubes

1 scoop vegan chocolate Shakeology powder

1 tbsp cacao nibs

2 tbsp soaked chia seeds (see page 268)

1 tbsp soaked almonds (see page 267) or almond butter

½ avocado

½ banana, 2 dates, or ¼ cup berries, for optional extra sweetener

Mix all ingredients in a blender or Vitamix until creamy.

*Makes 1 serving*

PER SERVING: 667 CALORIES, 35 G FAT, 71 G CARBS, 29 G PROTEIN

## *Lunch:*

### Kale and Seaweed Salad

8–10 large kale leaves, chopped

½ cup seaweed or 2 nori sheets cut in small squares

10 Sun Gold or other cherry or grape tomatoes, halved

½ red onion, minced

2 tbsp fresh mint and/or dill, chopped

1 tbsp cold-pressed extra-virgin olive oil

½ tsp apple cider vinegar

1 tsp mustard

Pinch of red pepper flakes

5 olives, pitted and chopped—Kalamata or other favorite

2 tbsp cashews (optional)

Place kale in a bowl. Add seaweed, tomatoes, onion, and mint.

For dressing, mix olive oil, cider vinegar, and mustard. Add to salad, toss, and top with olives and pepper flakes. Add cashews if desired, for an extra dose of protein.

PER SERVING: 408 CALORIES, 26 G FAT, 50 G CARBS, 8 G PROTEIN

## *Snack:*

### Easy Peel-and-Dip

1 banana
2 tbsp raw almond butter

Dip banana in almond butter.

PER SERVING: 301 CALORIES, 16 G FAT, 37 G CARBS, 37 G PROTEIN

## *Dinner:*

### Simple "Cheezy" Quinoa and Broccoli

1 cup sprouted quinoa
½ tsp Himalayan salt
1 tbsp coconut oil
2 cups broccoli, steamed
1 tbsp Bragg's Liquid Aminos or Coconut Secret Aminos
1 tbsp of nutritional yeast

Wash and cook quinoa according to package directions. Add Himalayan salt and coconut oil. Top with steamed broccoli and Bragg's, followed by nutrional yeast. Mix and eat.

*Makes 1 serving*

PER SERVING: 431 CALORIES, 56 G FAT, 53 G CARBS, 19 G PROTEIN
TOTAL DAILY VALUES: 1,807 CALORIES, 96 G FAT, 215 G CARBS, 66 G PROTEIN

# Day 6

*Breakfast:*

## Seasonal Fruit Bowl

½ cup raspberries

½ cup blackberries

½ cup strawberries

½ cup blueberries

½ tsp cinnamon powder

2 tbsp soaked chia seeds (see page 268)

Mix berries in bowl. Sprinkle cinnamon over them, and top with chia seeds.

*Makes 1 serving*

PER SERVING: 202 CALORIES, 10 G FAT, 28 G CARBS, 6 G PROTEIN

*Lunch:*

## "A Great Marriage" Quinoa and Kale

2 cups water

1 cup quinoa

1 cup broccoli

2 cups kale

1 tbsp coconut oil

½ avocado

½ tsp Himalayan salt

Wash and cook quinoa according to instructions on package.

Add kale and broccoli to cooked quinoa, and simmer 2–3 minutes more. If kale and broccoli need more time, take off simmer, cover pot, and let steam a bit longer.

Mix with coconut oil and avocado, and sprinkle with Himalayan salt.

*Makes 1 serving*

PER SERVING: 558 CALORIES, 31 G FAT, 65 G CARBS, 16 G PROTEIN*
ACCOMPANIED BY A RAW SALAD AT THAT MEAL, OR THAT DAY.

## *Snack:*

### Creamy Afternoon Pick-Me-Up Smoothie

½–1 cup coconut milk (see page 268)

½ cup fresh coconut water

4–5 ice cubes

2 tbsp soaked chia seeds

2 tbsp soaked cashews

½ tsp matcha green tea powder (or ½ cup brewed green tea, allowed to cool)

Toss all ingredients into a blender and blend until smooth.

PER SERVING: 580 CALORIES, 50 G FAT, 30 G CARBS, 13 G PROTEIN

## *Dinner:*

### Split Pea Soup

1 clove garlic, minced

1 medium yellow onion, chopped

1 tbsp avocado or coconut oil

1 tsp cumin

1 tbsp Bragg's Liquid Aminos or Coconut Secret Aminos

5 cups water

1 cup split peas

1 cup grated carrots

½ large sweet potato, chopped

1 tbsp pumpkin seeds

Sauté garlic and onion in avocado or coconut oil. Add cumin and aminos and blend well. Add water and split peas, bring to a boil, and simmer 2 minutes. Remove from heat, cover, and let sit for 1 hour.

Add remaining ingredients and simmer, covered, over low heat for about 2 hours. Adjust seasonings to taste. Add pumpkin seeds for garnish.

*Makes 2 servings*

PER SERVING: 353 CALORIES, 11 G FAT, 53 G CARBS, 14 G PROTEIN

TOTAL DAILY VALUES: 1,693 CALORIES, 101 G FAT, 175 G CARBS, 48 G PROTEIN

# Day 7

*Breakfast:*

## What a Blast Morning Smoothie

½ cup soaked almonds (see page 267)

1 tbsp raw cacao

½ avocado

1 banana

½ cup fresh basil leaves (as desired)

2 tbsp fresh mint leaves

8–12 ounces of water

3–4 ice cubes

Put water and ice in blender, then add the rest of the ingredients. Blend on high until smooth.

Almonds, cacao, and avocado are very rich, so use sparingly, depending on what your objective is. The mint and basil give this smoothie a nice taste while also increasing digestive potential. The rest of the ingredients are flavorful and dense in nutrients. Banana and avocado provide a creamy consistency. You can remove the cacao for a green morning smoothie.

*Makes 1 serving*

PER SERVING: 469 CALORIES, 31 G FAT, 50 G CARBS, 13 G PROTEIN

*Lunch:*

## Hummus Wrap

1 tbsp chopped red onion

½ cup each chopped green and red bell pepper

1 cup chopped shiitake mushrooms

10 oz store-bought organic roasted bell pepper or plain hummus

1 large or 2 small Ezekiel whole-grain tortillas

1 cup chopped fresh kale

½ avocado, sliced

½ cup cooked black beans (optional, for extra protein)

Mix onion, bell pepper, and mushroom with the hummus. Put on the tortilla with the kale, avocado, and black beans, if using. Roll into a wrap or burrito.

Eat raw, or warm in the oven or toaster oven at 200°F for 5–10 minutes.

*Makes 2 servings*

PER SERVING: 568 CALORIES, 24 G FAT, 69 G CARBS, 23 G PROTEIN

## *Snack:*

## Homemade Guaco-Love

2 medium avocados

PICO DE GALLO (MAKES APPROXIMATELY 1 CUP):

1 large ripe organic heirloom tomato, chopped

½ cup cilantro, roughly chopped

½ cup sweet onion, chopped

1 tbsp lime, peeled and chopped

1 jalapeño pepper, chopped

Smash avocados in a medium bowl. In a separate bowl, combine ingredients for pico de gallo. Serve mashed avocados with organic sprouted-corn tortilla chips, lightly toasted or raw (about 22), and ½ cup pico de gallo on the side.

*Makes 2 servings*

PER SERVING: 348 CALORIES, 25 G FAT, 32 G CARBS, 5 G PROTEIN

*Dinner:*

## Lentil Salad

1 cup dried lentils

1 cup diced carrots

½ cup diced red onions

⅓ cup thinly sliced green onions

2 cloves garlic, minced

1 bay leaf

½ tsp dried thyme

2 tbsp  freshly squeezed lemon juice

½ cup diced celery

½ cup chopped fresh cilantro

½ tsp Himalayan salt

½ tsp mixed dried herbs

½ cup avocado oil

In a saucepan combine lentils, carrots, onion, garlic, bay leaf, and thyme.

Add enough filtered or distilled water to cover by ½ inch. Bring to a boil, reduce heat, and simmer uncovered for 25 minutes, until lentils are tender but not mushy. Remove bay leaf.

Add avocado oil, lemon juice, celery, parsley, Himalayan salt, and mixed herbs.

Mix and serve at room temperature.

*Makes 2 servings*

PER SERVING: 427 CALORIES, 28 G FAT, 38 G CARBS, 10 G PROTEIN

TOTAL DAILY VALUES: 1,812 CALORIES, 108 G FAT, 188 G CARBS, 51 G PROTEIN

# Day 8

## *Breakfast:*

### Back to Life Fresh Smoothie

½ large frozen banana

3 frozen strawberries

½ cup fresh parsley (a handful)

½ cucumber, cut in pieces

1 cup unsweetened almond milk or coconut milk (see page 267)

Pinch cinnamon

2 tbsp freshly ground flaxseed

4 ice cubes

Note: if you can't freeze the fruit, add more ice cubes.

Put almond milk and ice in blender. Add the rest of the ingredients and blend until smooth.

*Makes 1 serving*

PER SERVING: 216 CALORIES, 10 G FAT, 32 G CARBS, 7 G PROTEIN

## *Lunch:*

### Tempeh Salad

4 oz tempeh, chopped into small cubes

½ cup organic chickpeas, cooked and rinsed (or substitute black beans)

½ cup shredded carrot

2 tbsp pumpkin seeds

½ tsp Himalayan salt

Mixed dried herbs or all-purpose seasoning (unsalted), to taste

2 tbsp chopped parsley, dill, basil, or cilantro

DRESSING (MAKES 2 SERVINGS)

3 tbsp Vegenaise (you can find it in any supermarket)*

2 tbsp French or Dijon mustard

2 tbsp soaked chia seeds (see page 268)

¼ cup apple cider vinegar

½ tsp Himalayan salt

Pinch paprika

Pinch mixed dried herbs or all-purpose seasoning (unsalted)

Toast tempeh in the oven for 5 minutes.

Put chickpeas or substitute tempeh, carrot, and seeds in a medium-sized bowl.

Whisk together all dressing ingredients until combined. Add ¼ cup of the dressing to salad, and toss. Add salt and mixed dried herbs to taste.

Finally, stir in fresh herbs, reserving a few to sprinkle on top.

*Makes 1 serving*

PER SERVING: 627 CALORIES, 32 G FAT, 53 G CARBS, 37 G PROTEIN

*Snack:*

## Almond Butter Heaven

½ cup almond butter

½ cup vanilla coconut milk—you can make your own coconut milk (see page 268) and flavor with vanilla

1 tbsp coconut sugar (agave or honey also works)

½ tsp cinnamon

A pinch Himalayan salt

1 green apple, sliced, or 4 stalks of celery (or substitute your favorite fruit or vegetable)

Blend first five ingredients until smooth. Transfer to a glass container and refrigerate 4 hours. Spread 4 tbsp on slices of apple or celery stalks.

*Makes 7 servings*

PER SERVING: 307 CALORIES, 21 G FAT, 23 G CARBS, 7 G PROTEIN

*Dinner:*

## Sweet Potato Soup

½ head cauliflower

2 pinches garam masala

1 tbsp coconut oil

1½ medium to large sweet potatoes, unpeeled, cut into 1-inch pieces

½ sweet onion, diced

1 clove garlic

3½ cups filtered water

½ tsp Himalayan salt

2 tbsp pine nuts or almonds

Preheat oven to 400°F.

Cut cauliflower into bite-size pieces and sprinkle lightly with garam masala. Spread cauliflower on ungreased cookie sheet and lightly drizzle with coconut oil. Place in preheated oven and roast until golden brown on the tops and tender, but not mushy, about 20–30 minutes. Remove and let rest.

In large stockpot, bring sweet potato, onion, garlic, and water to a boil. Add Himalayan salt and stir. Reduce heat and allow to remain at a constant simmer until sweet potatoes are tender. Add cooked cauliflower and divide soup into 2 equal parts. Let cool.

Blend half of the soup in blender until very smooth. Combine with unblended soup and stir. Season to taste with salt, and warm up on stovetop if needed.

Top with pine nuts or almonds.

*Makes 2 servings*

PER SERVING: 652 CALORIES, 28 G FAT, 92 G CARBS, 17 G PROTEIN

TOTAL DAILY VALUES: 1,802 CALORIES, 90 G FAT, 200 G CARBS, 68 G PROTEIN

# Day 9

## Breakfast:

### Morning Pudding

1 medium avocado

½ cup papaya, fresh if possible, frozen if not available

2 tbsp soaked chia seeds

½ cup coconut water, or substitute water kefir, almond milk, or raw milk

½ tbsp raw honey, or substitute yacon syrup, stevia, or agave to taste

Put all ingredients in a food processor or Vitamix, and pulse until smooth.

*Makes 1 serving*

PER SERVING: 441 CALORIES, 30 G FAT, 44 G CARBS, 10 G PROTEIN

## *Lunch:*

### Raw Lettuce Wraps

4 tbsp raw tahini or cashew paste

2 whole romaine lettuce leaves, large enough for making wraps

2 garlic cloves, pressed (roast first, if you wish)

1 tbsp shredded ginger

1 bell pepper, sliced in thin strips

1 medium zucchini or small jicama, sliced in thin strips

½ cup shredded carrot

½ cup sunflower sprouts or sprouts of choice

2 tbsp almonds, soaked, or peanuts, raw, or lightly toasted and crushed

Spread 2 tbsp tahini or cashew paste on each romaine leaf.

Layer the rest of the ingredients on top, dividing equally between the leaves, and wrap.

*Makes 2 wraps*

PER SERVING: 686 CALORIES, 30 G FAT, 52 G CARBS, 24 G PROTEIN

## *Snack:*

### Zinging Avocado Cacao Pudding

1 medium avocado, mashed

¼ cup raw, unsweetened 100 percent cacao powder

Pinch of cayenne powder

1½ tsp of honey or other sweetener

Combine ingredients in a bowl, and mash together.

*Makes 2 servings*

PER SERVING: 234 CALORIES, 13 G FAT, 25 G CARBS, 7 G PROTEIN

## *Dinner:*

### Wild Rice and Mushrooms

1 cup wild rice, cooked per instructions on package, or substitute quinoa, amaranth, alfalfa sprouts, radish sprouts, or broccoli

1 cup mushrooms, portobello or white preferred, cut up to desired size

2 tbsp chopped cilantro

1 medium heirloom tomato, chopped, or 4–5 cherry tomatoes, sliced

2 tbsp diced red onion

2 tbsp soaked almonds (see page 267), crushed or sliced into smaller pieces

Sea salt to taste

1–2 tbsp extra-virgin olive oil

Rinse and cook wild rice, or prepare alternative. Add mushrooms, cilantro, tomato, red onion, and almonds, if using. Season with sea salt, add olive oil, and mix to combine.

*Makes 1 serving*

PER SERVING: 639 CALORIES, 44 G FAT, 56 G CARBS, 17 G PROTEIN

TOTAL DAILY VALUES: 1,999 CALORIES, 135 G FAT, 177 G CARBS, 57 G PROTEIN

# Day 10

## *Breakfast:*

### Tempeh Breakfast Scramble

1 block three-grain organic tempeh (2 cups)

½ tsp onion powder

½ tsp Bragg's Liquid Aminos or Coconut Secret Aminos

½ tsp Himalayan salt

1½ tsp mixed dried herbs or all-purpose seasoning (unsalted)

½ tsp turmeric

½ tsp garlic powder

2 tbsp nutritional yeast flakes

In a medium bowl, mash tempeh with a fork until it looks like scrambled eggs. Add all other ingredients, and mix. Cook as you would scrambled eggs.

If you would like more texture, add a bit of coconut oil to a pan and sear the tempeh mixture at high temperature for 2–3 minutes.

*Makes 1–2 servings*

PER SERVING: 533 CALORIES, 18 G FAT, 49 G CARBS, 57 G PROTEIN

## *Lunch:*

### Red Quinoa Delight

2 tbsp goji berries or cranberries

1 cup quinoa, cooked (or substitute ½ cup soaked, crushed cashews, or use both)

1 red bell pepper, chopped

1 medium heirloom tomato

5 Kalamata olives, pitted

1 tbsp cold-pressed extra-virgin olive oil or coconut oil

1 tbsp chopped fresh basil

½ tsp Himalayan salt, or to taste

1 cucumber, peeled and chopped

2 tbsp nutritional yeast, plus a little to sprinkle on top

Use precooked quinoa, or wash and cook quinoa according to package instructions. While the quinoa is cooking, rehydrate goji berries in distilled water until plump. Drain extra water. Place berries in a bowl, add cooked quinoa and the remaining ingredients, and mix well.

Sprinkle top with nutritional yeast.

*Makes 1 serving*

PER SERVING: 642 CALORIES, 23 G FAT, 87 G CARBS, 23 G PROTEIN

## *Snack:*

## Berry Heaven

½ cup blueberries

½ cup raspberries

½ cup strawberries or pomegranate seeds

5 soaked walnuts

Mix and enjoy.

PER SERVING: 118 CALORIES, 5 G FAT, 18 G CARBS, 3 G PROTEIN

## *Dinner:* [Note: Please style as instructions.]

## Darin's Pizza

1 large Ezekiel sprouted-grain tortilla

2 tbsp fresh pesto or organic tomato paste

1 tbsp Vegenaise

⅓ cup quinoa (optional)

½ green pepper, sliced and diced

½ red pepper, sliced and diced

½ zucchini, sliced and diced

2 tbsp red onion, sliced and diced

1 tbsp basil

All-purpose seasoning (unsalted)

2 tbsp nutritional yeast, plus more to sprinkle on top

2 kale leaves

½ heirloom tomato, sliced

Lightly heat tortilla in oven, take out of oven, spread pesto or tomato paste on tortilla. Layer quinoa (if using), pepper, zucchini, onion, and basil over this; sprinkle with seasoning and nutritional yeast. Spread thin layer of Vegenaise, then add kale leaves and tomato. Sprinkle more nutritional yeast on top. Cook in conventional oven for 20–25 minutes at 325°F, or in dehydrator for 2 hours at 140°F, or 3 hours at 120°F.

PER SERVING: 650 CALORIES, 32 G FAT, 69 G CARBS, 20 G PROTEIN

TOTAL DAILY VALUES: 1,943 CALORIES, 78 G FAT, 223 G CARBS, 103 G PROTEIN

AVERAGE VALUES FOR TEN DAYS: 1,730 CALORIES, 94 G FAT, 188 G CARBS, 60 G PROTEIN

Some recipes for items to have on hand that you may not want to buy in the store:

## Soaked Almonds and Other Nuts

Cover raw organic almonds with distilled water and let soak overnight (8–12 hours). Rinse once or twice to eliminate anti-nutrients and starches and store in a glass container in the refrigerator.

## Ground flaxseed

Grind up flaxseed in a coffee grinder.

## Almond Milk

1 cup soaked almonds (see above), or other soaked nuts of your choice

4 cups water

1 tsp honey, stevia, yacon, or agave
½ tsp vanilla extract, cardamom, or cinnamon

Process water and almonds in a high-powered blender like a Vitamix. Strain first through a strainer and then through cheesecloth. (Leftover solids can be dehydrated and processed into a meal to use in gluten-free breads and so on.) Use immediately, or store in an air-tight glass container in the fridge.

You may do the same with walnuts, hazelnuts, Brazil nuts, or cashews.

## Coconut Milk

1 cup organic coconut shavings/flakes or dehydrated coconut strips
2 cups hot distilled water

Soak coconut in 2 cups hot water for every cup of coconut. Allow to sit in hot water until it cools to room temperature, and then transfer the mixture to a high-powered blender. Blend well, and then separate using a fine-mesh strainer or food-grade cheesecloth. Sweeten, salt, or add spices as desired. The leftover strained coconut solids can be used in gluten-free bread or many other recipes.

Using a fresh raw coconut (make sure it's ripe) is a lot more work, but the result is amazing. Cut the top of the coconut carefully in a circle, and pop that piece out. Drain the coconut water into the blender. Scrape as much meat as possible from the inside of the coconut, and add that to the blender. Blend on high, strain, and add flavor if you wish.

## Soaked Chia Seeds

To 4 cups of distilled water in a glass pitcher or jar, add 5 tbsp organic chia seeds. Shake once, let sit for 1 minute, shake again, and put in the fridge. Use after 8–12 hours, when it has taken on a gel-like consistency. It will keep in the fridge up to a week.

Use in salads and smoothies over the week, or combine with the juice of ½ organic orange in a glass as a drink.

# Darin's Daily Simple Fixes

Health is created one choice at a time. It really is that simple! Once you know what healthy choices to make, you repeat them over and over again. That's how health becomes a lifestyle. Here you'll find a list of my favorite fixes and ones that will have the greatest impact on your health. Pick a simple fix on this list—any fix!—and get started. Whether you work through them in order or jump around, the key is to pick something that resonates with you. Keep making one simple change at a time and you'll arrive at a healthy lifestyle before you know it!

- Drink at least half an ounce of water per pound of body weight but closer to your body weight in ounces (a 120-pound person should drink a minimum of sixty ounces of water daily, or around half a gallon). Add half a teaspoon of unrefined crystal salt, like Himalayan salt, to each gallon.

- When you drink your water, vortate it, love it, and structure it. It will work better in the body that way. Water is sensitive!

- Cut way down on meat, fish, eggs, and dairy, eating them only once or twice a week at most, and even then in small portions. Make sure your beef is grass-fed, your fish wild-caught, your eggs organic and free-range, and your dairy grass-fed and unpasteurized whenever possible.

- Drink green tea.

- Eat organic berries, fresh or frozen.

- Eat raw leafy greens every day, the darker the better.

- Seek out fermented foods like kimchi, sauerkraut, miso, and tempeh.

- Replace pasteurized cow's milk and cheese with fermented kefir or raw yogurt.

- Eat almonds, almond butter, and almond milk. Remember to sprout and soak!

- Eat cruciferous vegetables—broccoli, broccoli sprouts, cauliflower, Brussels sprouts, cabbage.

- Eat cold-pressed plant fats such as olive, sasha inchi, coconut, avocado oil, and fair-trade palm oil. Even organic raw butter is a lot better than most vegetable oils.

- Chew more. Slow meals down.

- Avoid bread, pasta, crackers, or anything else made with white flour or any other refined wheat products.

- Avoid not only sugar itself but also concentrated sweeteners like corn syrup, as well as artificial sweeteners, which are even worse than sugar. Shoot for 10 grams or less of added sugar per meal.

- Eliminate processed foods, which means anything that somebody else has prepared—unless it's somebody who loves you. Eat whole foods!

- Avoid soda, concentrated fruit juice, energy drinks, and sports drinks.

- Turn the bad old traditional food pyramid upside down: make plants the biggest portion of your daily eating.

- Before you eat, stop, take a deep breath, and express some gratitude. We have so much to be grateful for.

- Stop eating when you feel 80 percent full. In ten minutes you will feel totally satisfied. It's better for your health.

- Take full responsibility for your health. Doctors are smart about sickness, but nobody teaches them how to keep us well. That's your job!

- Don't use other people and their habits as an excuse for eating badly. What you put in your mouth is your decision alone.

- Don't whine. If you don't like something, change it or don't, but act as though it's your decision—because it is. It's your life. Don't give it away!

- Eat huge salads filled with leafy greens, other vegetables, sprouts, beans, fruit, seeds, and nuts. Use a really big bowl. Eat a lot. Every day!

- Put natural fibers—organic cotton, linen, silk, wool, hemp—next to your skin. It's your biggest organ, and deserves more respect than most people give it. Rubbing all day against a petroleum-based clothing product is doing you no favors.

- Eat half or more of your vegetables and fruit raw.

- Stop buying products from companies that don't care whether they're making us sick.

- Act like you feel lucky to be alive. Your body will work better, and probably so will your life!

- Have great sex without Viagra or any other pharmaceutical assistance. If you need a little help, try all the Life Forces first as well as natural plant cures. There are many!

- Breathe a lot, all the way in and all the way out. Breathing with your nose is one of the best stress reductions you can perform.

- Avoid daily coffee. You only think you need it. There are much healthier sources of energy. Remember, it is very acidic, which outweighs any other benefits.

- Only acquire good habits—a lot of them. If you're gonna do things over and over again, you might as well do things that help you, not hurt you.

- Wear fewer clothes—expose yourself to the sun and air. The light and vitamin D are good for you. Leave off the sunscreen so the sun can get in. (Of course, be careful not to burn yourself.)

- Go barefoot—shoes weaken the muscles in your feet and keep you from feeling the earth. Even better, go barefoot outdoors so you can feel the planet's vibration, which is beneficial to your health. Walk on grass or dirt or sand, take a hike, ride a wave, climb a rock, hug a tree, reconnect to the forces that made us.

- Pay attention to and be outside for the sunrise or sunset. It activates the brain!

- Lift heavy things, whether at the gym or at home, whether you're a man or a woman. It releases growth hormones and testosterone, which are good for us.

- Eat an avocado.

- Allow yourself to feel chilly—turn on the cold water for the last thirty seconds of every shower, jump in a cold lake or ocean, go outside on a cool day in a T-shirt and shorts. A little chill pumps the capillaries, increases fat burning, stimulates the immune system, and keeps you young.

- Eat some nutrient-dense, powerful superfoods: mushrooms, moringa, kale . . . Find some new ones, too.

- Avoid anything with artificial fragrances—soap, shampoo and other hair products, deodorant, perfumes, cosmetics, laundry detergents. These chemicals just add to the toxic stew our immune systems already have to deal with. If you need a scent, use an essential oil, like lavender, rose, frankincense, and sandalwood, which will boost your mood and increase pH.

- Eat nuts—germinated, if possible, since that makes them less acidic, more nutritious, and better for your digestion.

- Eat seeds and pseudograins such as quinoa, chia seeds, and flaxseed. Humans have been eating seeds and some grains for over 40,000 years.

- Shoot for an 70/30 mix—70 percent fresh, whole plant foods, 30 percent everything else (except unhealthy foods, of course).

- Sleep in total darkness—that means no phone, no clock, no iPad or TV, and no outside light coming in through the curtains. Use an eye pillow if you need to.

- Just get outside every day and move, walk, work, work out, play, and breathe.

- Listen! Listen to yourself, your knowing, your inner environment. By doing this, you honor yourself. Some forms of meditation, such as stopping, are extremly beneficial to your health.

- Avoid fried food, especially if it's been fried in something nasty, unnatural, or unknown. This includes nearly every kind of chip, pretzel, and other prepared snack food.

- Eat brightly colored vegetables, lightly steamed, roasted, or sautéed.

- Laugh. Play. Get together with people you like.

- Try a new fruit or veggie every week. Diversification is a major key to optimal health. And don't forget your superfoods!

# Acknowledgments

We are not alone in this life. We may decide to create something but we are never alone in that creation. We are inspired by each other. I know I am, supported and guided as well as constantly learning from others. All that we do is in some way because of someone else. We are not alone, ever.

My father, Howard Olien, was such a big influence on me, encouraging me when I struggled and always trying to teach me to work hard. He allowed me enough freedom to figure things out, enabling me to discover what was important to me both physically as an athlete and as a man. Dad, I miss you and love you every day. Thanks for your guidance. Rest in peace. Mom, Sandy Olien, you loved me and did anything and everything you could so that I felt loved and taken care of throughout my life. I noticed everything you did, and all that loving and caring has allowed me to love myself totally, which in turn has enabled me to share, care, and help others. I love you. To my older brother, Troy, I am happy to be a part of your life and of the lives of your family, Julee, Logan, and Hanna. To Jenna and Nathan Olien, my other brother and sister from my dad's second marriage, we are forever connected through him. You amaze and inspire me with your beyond-your-years curiosity and interest in learning. I love you. And to Deb Schmidt-Olien, for doing everything you can to raise some amazing kids in spite of tremendous challenges. I don't see you all often enough, but you are always in my heart.

I also thank:

All the older guys in the weight room in my hometown of Waseca, Minnesota, who first taught me about lifting and working out.

My high school and college coaches and teammates for letting me do something with all this energy I had.

Tony Anderson, for pushing me in the weight room when I no longer had football as an outlet. Your close friendship and ridiculous strength were always such a motivation to me.

Tyrone Stenzel, for teaching me and letting me assist you as strength coach back in the days at the University of St. Thomas.

Dale Greenwald. Fresh out of college, I showed up in Boulder, Colorado, ready to help people with nutrition, fitness, and health, and it would not have been the same had I not met an amazing man who was carving his own way in helping and rehabbing people. Dale, thank you for mentoring me, for letting me be your partner for all those years, and for teaching me about proper movement. You not only helped me, but allowed me to help hundreds of people.

Ted Waitkus, because you believed in me and encouraged me when I was fresh and naive. I can't tell you how much your friendship has meant to me.

Pharmacist Ben Fuchs. Your wisdom and entrepreneurial spirit inspired me to think outside the box and get back to letting the body heal itself. It was fun to start educating others and selling supplements with you before anyone else was really doing that.

Dr. Bob Stilson, the private lectures and research articles you gave me about natural health and nutrition encouraged me and showed me that I was on the right path of fueling the body with herbs and whole foods.

Ariel and Kristin Solomon, you were and still are an extension of my family. All those miles on the Harleys and all those heavy weights trying to keep up with your NFL strength were inspiring.

Barb and Bob Holzer, thank you for letting me live with you for those formative years in Colorado. Barb, your spiritual guidance influenced one of the most significant times in my life. I miss you. Rest in peace.

My adopted Colorado family, Steve Devanney, Sarah Jane Geraldi, Raven-Sky, and River. Stevie, you and I bonded through our motorcycle road trips and are connected through the heart. Thanks for flying with me and helping me discover who I am. I love what we shared and share, brother! Sarah Jane Geraldi, your depth of caring and connection is awe-inspiring and your light has been a huge gift to me and to your family. Raven-Sky, being your godparent has been one of the greatest gifts ever. I watched you being born, and from that day you have blessed my life as I watched you become a woman. You are a powerful light. River, I am proud to be your godparent. As I watched you being born swimming in a pool in the living room, I knew you were going to be different, the kind of difference that can change the world.

Lauren Monroe, Rick Allen, and Josie my goddaughter, your love and caring have allowed me to see way beyond myself and contribute more to others and to the planet.

Dr. Mohsen Hourmanesh, you inspired and educated me on nutrition and living healthy more than any single person. You are one of the most brilliant and generous people I know, with a loving heart and desire for the truth.

Randall Masters, if not for the private gatherings in your home, with some of the smartest people on the planet, I would not see the things I see now. Your lectures on color, sound, mathematics, and frequencies were and are way ahead of their time.

Mark Sisson, for believing in me when I was creating some of my first formulas and mentoring me with your knowledge and encouragement. I am proud of what you are creating.

To my friends and workout "boys" in Malibu. Words can't express how wonderful it is to have a group of buddies like you. Laird Hamilton and Gabby Reece, I am so very grateful to you for opening your hearts and home to me, creating a meeting place for all of us to better ourselves, to be inspired and contribute. To the boys with whom I spend nearly every day pushing on, sweating, supporting, playing, and becoming stronger, I have become a better man and person from all your contributions. We have a special group that is greater than the sum of its parts. Thanks, Hutch Parker, Johnny McGinley, Sam Sumyk, Dave Anawalt, Max Musina, Chris Gough, Rick Rubin, Randy Wallace, Tom Jones and all the other guys who come and go.

A chance encounter with Carl and Isabelle Daikeler changed my professional life forever. Isabelle, you have become such a good friend in the process of our finding how to approach health and nutrition. Carl, your faith in me from the beginning to create Shakeology was one of the greatest professional expressions I have ever witnessed. You trusted me, respected me, and gave me the space to create. I have learned so much from both of you and look forward to an even greater future of helping people make healthy choices the norm rather than the exception.

To the many people at Beachbody I have worked with, I can't possible thank everyone. However, some of the people I have been touched by are Jon Congdon, Jonathan Gelfand, Carolina Gutinsky, Nancy Marcello, Mike Wilson, Marc Washington, Phillipa Bernstine, Lisa Lyons, Carrie Dobro, Tony Horton, Steve Edwards, Richard Andrew, Dana Brown, David Reece, Pamela Keller, Maria Angeli, Kay Duncan, Sandi Bouhadana, May Lam, Miguel Amezcua, Keith Harris, Aaron Morton, and many others.

Seth Tuckerman, I'm in awe of your integrity and business sense. The many miles we have traveled and the lessons I have learned from you have been priceless. We really gave it a go, and you helped me to help the farmers and keep the integrity of quality superfoods.

Robert Plarr, a renegade spirit in the conscious environmental movement, way before those terms even existed, forty years ago. You inspire me with your relentless pursuit of a better life for all people.

Adam Good, your friendship has been steady and true and your passion and heart are always in the right place.

Chris Patton, one of the most fun, fascinating, and action-positive people I know. I have no doubt that what you are creating will make a positive change in the world.

Craig and Maria Cooper, you have been an inspiration over the last few years in how to live fully and care for and be true to ourselves.

Bernd Neugebauer, your wisdom of plants, biodynamics, fermentation, and sustainable and indigenous farming has touched and influenced me forever. I bow to the wonderful connection we have.

Who thanks their lawyer? Well, I do! Lee Sacks, you have been a great adviser, watching over my affairs with professionalism and keen understanding, and an even greater friend, and that combination helps me feel guided and protected.

Bruce Kolbrener, for believing in me early on, educating me and advising me about my money and finances. Your wisdom, professionalism, and guidance have helped me out of fear of money and into total abundance.

To my team! You help me manifest my dreams to help people live healthy and abundant lives. Miguel Beruman, our shared vision of being true to ourselves and the indigenous people and farmers started much of this. Your knowledge, passion, and desire to help others are what connected us and keep us at it to this day. Linda Zielski, your years of dedication and belief in hard work are so very important to me, not to menton the amazingly loving person you are. David Zielski, for years of relentless work and dedication in all the ventures we have been involved in, especially the place you have taken our nonprofit organizaton, RainCatcher. org, getting kids clean water around the world. Hiram Santiteban, for bringing your knowledge, wisdom, and bright spirit to me and the Superlife team. Your desire to help, inspire, and uplift people is a perfect fit.

To the greatest love of my life, my beloved woman and wife, Eliza Coupe. Your coming into my life has been my single greatest discovery and blessing! You make me a better man. I celebrate the brilliance and beauty you are. I can't even begin to utter the level of respect, love, and care I have for you. You are my family, my friend, my partner, and the love I have always desired. I love you totally.

And to all the other healers, doctors, researchers, farmers, producers, and explorers in all the other countries and continents I have met along the Superfood hunting trail: Thank you for teaching me, housing me, hosting me, and sharing your wisdom so that together we can contribute to a healthier planet and people.

And a special thanks to the book team, Bill Tonelli for your contribution and writing mastery. I could not have done this without you. To my agent, Richard Pine, thanks for bringing in your expertise and experience to this project. Thank you, Sara Brady, for research assistance. And thank you to the amazing publishing team at Harper Wave. Karen Rinaldi, you are one of the greats. If not for how wonderful you are and how easy you made the process, this book would not have happened. And thank you to the rest of the Harper team for believing in this kid from Minnesota who has a desire to contribute to the world in a healthy way.

# Appendix A: The Big Acid-Alkaline List

## ALKALINE-FORMING FOODS
### (FRESH FOODS ARE GENERALLY MORE ALKALIZING)

Alfalfa sprouts
All melons
Apple cider vinegar
Apples
Apricots
Artichokes
Arugula
Asparagus
Avocado
Baking powder
Baking soda
Basil
Beans (fresh, green)
Beets
Black berries
Blueberries
Bok Choy
Cabbage
Cantaloupe
Cashews
Cauliflower
Celery
Chestnuts
Chia seeds
Cinnamon
Coconut water (fresh)
Collard greens
Cumin
Dandelion greens
Dill
Eggplant
Fruit juices (only fresh)
Garlic

Ginger root (fresh)
Ginseng tea
Grapefruit
Grapefruit juice
Grapes
Grapes (sweet)
Green onions
Herbs (fresh)
Herbs (leafy green)
Himalaya Salt
Honeydew
Kale
Kelp
Kimchi
Kiwi fruits
Kombucha
Lemon juice
Lemons
Lettuce (most)
Limes
Mandarins
Mango
Marjoram
Mint
Miso
Molasses (unsulfured
Nectarine
Onions
Oranges
Oregano
Papaya
Paprika
Parsley

Parsnips
Pears
Peppers
Pineapple
Pineapple juice
Pumpkin seeds
Radish
Raisins
Raspberry
Red pepper flakes
Rosemary
Salad greens
Sea salt
Sea vegetables
Seaweeds
Spices
Spirulina
Strawberries
Sweet potato
Tamari
Tangerine
Thyme
Turnip
Vegetable juices (fresh)
Water (fresh spring)
Watercress
Yams
Zucchini

## NEUTRAL FOODS

Almond butter
Almonds
Apple juice (fresh)
Avocado oil
Berry juice (fresh)
Bragg's Aminos
Brown rice vinegar
Brussel sprouts
Buckwheat (flour)
Carrots (organic)
Cayenne pepper
Chamomile tea
Cilantro
Coconut (meat, young, fresh)
Coconut butter
Coconut oil
Cucumber
Fava beans

Flax seed
Flax seed oil
Ghee
Grape juice (fresh)
Hemp seed oil
Honey (raw)
Jicama
Macadamia
Millet
Mushrooms
Oats (steel cut)
Olive oil (extra virgin)
Orange juice (Fresh)
green tea
Peas (fresh)
Pickles (homemade)
Potatoes (with skin)
Primrose oil
Quinoa

Rice syrup
Rooibos
Sake
Sauerkraut
Seeds (most)
Sesame seeds (whole)
Soy beans
Soy sauce
Sprouted grains
Sprouts
Sunflower seeds
Tahini (raw)
Tempeh
Tomatoes
Wild rice
Yeast (nutritional flakes)
Yerba mate

## ACID-FORMING FOODS
## (MEAT AND PROCESSED FOODS ARE ACIDIC)

Aspartame
Bananas (green)
Barley
Bran
Butter (conventional)
Cacao (conventional)
Casein
Cereals (unrefined)
Cheese
Chestnut oil
Chicken liver
Chicken meat
Coffee (decaf)
Corn (canned, processed)
Cow milk (whole)
Crackers (unrefined rye,

rice and wheat)
Cranberries
Cream cheese
Duck
Egg yolks (soft cooked)
Eggs whole (hard cooked)
Fish
Goat's milk (homogenized)
Milk protein
Granola
Ham
Maple syrup (processed)
Oat bran
Olives (ripe)
Palm kernel oil

Peanut butter
Peanut oil
Peanuts
Pecans
Pistachios
Pomegranate
Rice milk
Rye
Scallops
See dairy
Soybean oil
Squid
Turkey
Wheat bread (sprouted organic)
Wheat germ
Whole grain tortillas

## Other:

Lard
Mayonnaise

Mustard
Ketchup

Tapioca

## ALKALIZING ACTIONS

Love
Kindness
Peace
Prayer
Meditation

Exercise/movement
Breathing deeply (oxygen)
Gratitude
Giving

## ACIDIFYING ACTIONS

| | | |
|---|---|---|
| Overwork | Stress | Lack of sleep |
| Fear | Resentment | Fighting |
| Anger | Overtraining/ | |
| Jealousy | overexercise | |

# Appendix B: Sources

## SUPERFOODS

Shakeology
Navitas Naturals
Sambazon

Big Tree Farms
Earth Sift Products
Surthrival

Vivapura
Longevity Warehouse

## HERBS AND SPICES

Mountain Rose Herbs

Frontier Coop

Sand Mountain Herbs

## FARMS AND MARKETS

USDA Farmers Market
  Search

Local Harvest
Fruits, veggies, all food

## SOURCES

### Superfoods

www.SuperLifeShake.
  com
www.navitasnaturals.com
www.sambazon.com

www.bigtreefarms.com
www.earthshiftproducts.
  com
www.surthrival.com

www.vivapura.com
www.longevitywarehouse
  .com

### Herbs and Spices

www.mountainroseherbs
  .com

www.frontiercoop.com

www.sandmountainherbs
  .com

### Farms and Markets

http://search.ams.usda
  .gov/farmersmarkets/
www.localharvest.org
local farmers market,

organic local health
food market or store

**PRODUCT**

## Superfoods

Moringa
Cacao powder
Cacao nibs
Chlorella
Nutritional yeast
Chia
Nuts

Dried coconut
Frozen organic coconut
   water
Maca
Goji berries
Fermented foods

Make your own
   fermented foods
Nori seaweed sheets
Sprouted seeds
Spirulina chrystalized
Inca berries

## Sweeteners

Coconut sugar
Raw honey

Stevia
Yacon syrup

Agave

## Spices/Condiments

Vanilla extract
Spices
Cardamom

Cinnamon
Garam marsala
Apple cider vinegar

Tamarind paste
Liquid aminos

## Butters/Oils

Cashew butter
Coconut butter
Coconut oil

Almond butter
Mesquite powder
All-season herb

Himalayan salt
Tahini

## Grains

Tempeh
Teff/fonio
Oats

Quinoa
Tortilla, sprouted
Tortilla corn, sprouted

Bread, sprouted

## Supplements

Shakeology (meal
   replacement)

Ultimate reset (21-day
   cleanse)

## Vertical Grow Systems

Verti Farms

Living Tower

## Garden

Small space gardens

Seeds

Pests

# BRANDS

## SUPERFOODS

Moringa Source
Sunu Harvest
Big Tree Farms
Z Natural Foods
Viva Pura
Navitas Naturals

Wilderness Family
  Naturals
Exotic Superfoods
Dragon Herbs
Rejuvenative
Cultures for Health

Maine Coast
Emeral Cove
Go Raw
Raw Guru

## Sweeteners

Big Tree Farms
Local farmer

Sweetleaf
Ojio

Navitas Naturals
Ojio

## Spices/Condiments

Frontier
Bragg's

Aunt Patty's Coconut
  Secret

## Butters/Oils

Artisana
Nutiva
Living Tree Community

Navitas Naturals
Simply Organic
Himala

Viva Pura

## Grains

Light Life
Bob's Red Mill

To Your Health Sprouted
Ezekiel 4:9

## Supplements

www.SuperLifeShake.com    www.ultimatereset.com

## Vertical Grow Systems

http://growvertigarms.com    www.livingtowers.com

## Garden

www.woollypocket.com
www.seedsavers.org
http://cottagegardener
  .com

www.earthworkshealth
  .com

## WEBSITES

### *Superfoods*

www.moringasource.com
http://organic-moringa
  .com
www.bigtreefarms.com
www.znaturalfoods.com
www.vivapura.com
http://navitasnaturals
  .com

# Index

# About the Author

**DARIN OLIEN** is an exotic superfood hunter, supplement formulator, environmental activist, and widely recognized authority on nutrition and natural health. He partnered with the fitness company Beachbody to formulate the wildly popular whole-food supplement Shakeology and the comprehensive plant-based Ultimate Reset 21-day detoxification program. He also sits on the board of Raincatcher.org, a nonprofit dedicated to providing clean drinking water. He holds a BA in exercise physiology/nutrition and an MA in psychology, and lives in Malibu, California.